Everyone Owns Safety

A Pocket Guide to Every Function's Role in Medical Device Risk Management

PUBLISHED BY: Pujitha Gourabathini

Print ISBN: 979-8-9959804-9-0
eBook ISBN: 979-8-9959804-4-5

Published by **Pujitha Gourabathini**
First Edition, 2026

This book is for educational purposes only. It does not constitute professional regulatory, legal, or clinical advice. Readers should consult applicable standards, regulations, and qualified professionals when making decisions related to medical device safety or compliance.

Printed in the United States of America

www.linkedin.com/in/pujitha-gourabathini/

Dedication

To my mentors who shaped my thinking — within my company and across the medical device industry — thank you for the guidance, the inspiration, the questions that pushed me further, and the wisdom that helped bring this book to life.

To my family, whose steady encouragement, support and patience carried me through the long hours required to bring this first book to completion.

Acknowledgments

With gratitude to the LTR Risk Coach, an AI-powered risk-leadership thinking partner for MedTech QA/RA, R&D, Clinical, and Risk professionals, whose support helped shape and strengthen the ideas in this book.

Table of Contents

Preface

Over the course of my career in the medical device industry, I have seen firsthand how product safety and risk management are often treated as specialized activities carried out by a small group of experts. These teams work diligently to create and maintain the risk management file—an essential document intended to guide risk-based decisions throughout the product lifecycle. Yet in practice, many functions across an organization are unaware that this file exists, unclear about how it should inform their daily work, or unsure of their own role in contributing to patient safety.

This gap is not due to lack of commitment. It is due to lack of clarity.

Every function—whether technical, operational, clinical, or commercial—interacts with health and safety risk in meaningful ways. Each one generates inputs that shape the risk management file and relies on outputs from it to make informed, responsible decisions. But without a shared understanding of how these connections work, organizations unintentionally create silos that weaken the very systems designed to protect patients.

This pocket guide was written to close that gap. It is not a technical manual, nor is it a regulatory textbook. Instead, it is a practical, accessible reference for professionals across all functions in a medical device organization. Its purpose is simple: to illuminate how each role contributes to product safety, how each function interacts with risk, and how the risk management file can serve as a central point of reference for the decisions made every day.

My hope is that this guide brings clarity, strengthens cross-functional alignment, and reinforces a shared commitment to patient safety—because risk management is not the responsibility of a select few. It is the responsibility of all of us.

Introduction

Medical devices exist to improve health, restore function, and protect life. With that purpose comes an obligation: every decision made within a medical device organization must consider its impact on patient safety. Risk management is the framework that enables this responsibility. It provides a disciplined approach to identifying, evaluating, controlling, and monitoring risk throughout the product lifecycle.

Yet despite its importance, risk management is often misunderstood as a specialized activity owned by a single team. In reality, it is a system that depends on contributions from every function. Engineering, quality, clinical affairs, regulatory, manufacturing, supply chain, marketing, customer service, post-market surveillance, and many others—all influence the safety profile of a device. Each function makes decisions that carry risk implications, and each one relies on information contained in the risk management file.

This book is designed to make those connections clear.

It provides a concise overview of the major functions within a medical device organization and describes how each one interacts with health and safety risk. It outlines the inputs each function provides to the risk management file, the outputs they depend on, and the types of risk-based decisions they make in their daily responsibilities. The goal is not to teach the technical details of ISO 14971 or regulatory requirements, but to offer a practical, easy-to-use reference that helps professionals at all stages of their careers, from new engineers to experienced leaders, to understand their role in maintaining and strengthening patient safety.

Whether you are new to the industry, transitioning into a new function, or seeking to deepen your understanding of how your work contributes to the broader safety system, this guide is intended to support you. By fostering shared understanding and cross-functional alignment, organizations can build stronger, more resilient safety cultures—where risk management is not a document, but a culture and way of thinking.

PART I — The Foundation: What Risk Management Actually Is

Chapter 1: Risk Is Not a Document; It Is a Decision

What Risk Management Actually Is — And What It Is Not

Risk management is one of the most misunderstood activities in the medical device industry. It is often treated as a document, a template, a file to be completed, reviewed, and archived. But risk management is not a document. It is not a formality, a deliverable, or a milestone. It is not something that exists only during design and development or something that is "owned" by a single function.

Risk management is a decision-making framework. It is the disciplined practice of asking — at every stage of a device's life — what can go wrong, how badly it can go wrong, how likely it is, and what will be done about it. Every answer to those questions is a decision. Every decision has consequences. And in medical devices, those consequences reach patients.

Over time, organizations have built processes that resemble well-functioning safety systems: templates, checklists, procedures, and documentation that look complete and compliant. People are trained to produce these outputs on time. But somewhere along the way, the focal point of these efforts can be forgotten — the patient, the clinical user, the individual who relies on the device being safe.

This creates a specific kind of false confidence. A risk management file that is extensive, properly formatted, and fully signed can give the impression that safety has been thoroughly considered. It satisfies auditors. It checks the box for project teams. But it does not guarantee that the right decisions were made with the right inputs at the right time.

This leads directly to the misconception at the center of the problem.

The Misconception at the Center of Everything

Across the industry, one belief is so common and so deeply embedded that it shapes how organizations operate:

Risk management is what the risk team is responsible for.

It is understandable why this belief exists. Most organizations have a function — often within Quality or Regulatory — that maintains the risk management file, produces hazard analyses, and interfaces with regulators. That function has specialized expertise. It owns the tools and the procedures. When something touches risk, people go to that function. The conclusion seems logical: risk management is their job.

But risk management cannot be siloed. It is not a specialty. It is a property of decisions — and decisions are made by everyone.

The person who writes the intended use statement is making a risk decision. The engineer who changes a requirement is making a risk decision. The manufacturing engineer who adjusts a process step is making a risk decision. The project manager who accelerates a schedule is making a patient safety decision. The complaint handler who codes a field report is making a risk decision.

None of these individuals may think of their work in those terms. But if a decision affects what the device does, how it performs, who uses it, or the conditions under which it operates — it is a risk decision. And it belongs inside the risk management framework, not adjacent to it. This misunderstanding leads to another challenge.

The False Confidence Problem

A risk management file created with genuine rigor looks almost identical to one created simply to satisfy a procedural checkpoint. Both have the correct structure. Both use the standard terminology. Both appear complete.

The difference does not appear in the file itself. It appears downstream.

It appears when a complaint describes a failure mode that was never anticipated because the hazard analysis was finalized too early and never revisited. It appears when a design change unintentionally alters a risk control because no one connected the change to the risk file. It appears when post-market data reveals a pattern that contradicts the assumptions made during development.

This is how a poorly executed risk management process becomes a patient safety risk in its own right — not through dramatic failures, but through the quiet accumulation of decisions made in the shadow of documentation that looks like safety assessment but does not deliver it.

To understand how this happens, it helps to see how risk decisions are distributed across the organization.

How This Connects Across the Organization

Every function in a medical device company makes decisions that influence patient safety. Some decisions are obvious — design choices, verification strategies, clinical evaluations. Others are subtle — coding a complaint, adjusting a process parameter, interpreting a supplier change, or approving a schedule.

Each chapter that follows is dedicated to one of these functions. It will introduce you to the decisions that function makes, the safety implications of those decisions, and the role that function plays in shaping the risk management file.

The purpose is not to turn every employee into a risk expert. It is to give every person the clarity they need to recognize when they are making a risk-relevant decision — and to understand how to make that decision with the right information, at the right time, with the right mindset.

This leads to the single idea at the heart of this book.

The One Thing This Book Is Asking of You

Risk management is difficult not because the methodology is complex, but because misconceptions persist: that risk management is a document, that it is owned by Quality, that it happens only during development, that a signed hazard analysis proves a device is safe.

These misconceptions exist because many people were never given a clear picture of what risk management actually is, what it requires, and why it matters.

Every decision made during the development, manufacture, and post-market life of a medical device is, in some sense, a product risk decision — a choice that shapes what the device does, how reliably it does it, and how safely it can be used by the people who need it.

That is the single idea this book is built on. Every chapter that follows is an application of it — to your function, your decisions, your conversations, your work.

The patient at the center of your work is counting on all of it.

Notes & Sources

- **On risk management as a lifecycle discipline rather than a documentation activity —** ISO 14971:2019, *Medical devices — Application of risk management to medical devices*, Clause 4. International Organization for Standardization.
- **On manufacturer-level responsibility for safety —** FDA Quality Management System Regulation (21 CFR Part 820, effective February 2026), which harmonizes with ISO 13485:2016. U.S. Food and Drug Administration, *Quality Management System Regulation*, 21 CFR Part 820, 2024.

Chapter 2: What Safety Risk Management Actually Means

The Bicycle

In the last chapter, we established that risk management is not merely a document. It is a decision-making framework — a systematic way of asking what can go wrong, how badly, how likely, and what to do about it.

Before you can make those decisions well, you need a vocabulary. Not the kind of vocabulary that requires a dictionary to navigate. The kind that, once you have it, makes the logic of the whole system click into place.

That vocabulary comes from ISO 14971 — the international standard that governs risk management for medical devices. It has precise definitions for terms that sound familiar but mean something specific in this context. And those precise definitions matter, because when people use them loosely, or interchangeably, or incorrectly, the risk analysis itself becomes unreliable in ways that are not always visible until something goes wrong in the field.

This chapter is going to give you that vocabulary — all of it in plain language. Using a bicycle.

Not because medical devices are like bicycles. But because the concepts of risk management are universal — they apply to anything that has the potential to cause harm to a person — and a bicycle is something everyone understands intuitively. Once the concept clicks in a context you already know, translating it to the medical device world becomes straightforward.

So, you have a bicycle. Let us talk about risk.

Hazard

A hazard is anything that ***has the potential to cause harm***.

On your bicycle, there are several hazards. The chain is one — if something gets caught in it while you are riding, it could pull you off balance. The wheels are another — moving at speed, they can cause serious injury in a collision. The frame, if it fails, could send you to the ground without warning. None of these things are hurting anyone right now. The bicycle is sitting in your garage, perfectly still, perfectly quiet. But the potential for harm is present in each of them. That potential is what makes them hazards.

Notice what a hazard is not. It is not the harm itself. It is not the event that causes the harm. It is the underlying source — the thing that, under the right circumstances, could hurt someone. The chain does not have to actually catch a shoelace to be a hazard. It is a hazard whether or not any shoelace ever comes near it.

This distinction matters more than it might seem. In medical device organizations, hazards are frequently confused with failure modes or malfunctions or defects. An engineer analyzing a device failure might identify the failure as "motor stops unexpectedly" and treat that as the hazard. But the motor stopping unexpectedly is not a hazard. It is an event. The hazard — the underlying source of potential harm — might be the kinetic energy of a moving component that is no longer controlled, or the interruption of a therapy that a patient depends on. Getting this wrong means the risk control gets aimed at the wrong target. The motor failure gets addressed, but the underlying hazard that the motor failure exposes may not.

Why this matters: If you misidentify the hazard, every downstream risk control will be aimed at the wrong target.

In medical devices, hazards take many forms: electrical energy, mechanical force, biological or chemical substances, radiation, incorrect information delivered to a clinical user, or software behavior that controls a therapy. The first job of risk management is to identify them — completely, systematically, and without assuming that a device with no failures has no hazards. Every medical device has hazards.

Hazardous Situation

Once you understand the hazard, the next question is: **when does a person actually become exposed to it?**

A hazardous situation is the moment when a person — a patient, a clinical user, a bystander — is exposed to a hazard.

Back to your bicycle. The chain, as we established, is a hazard. It sits there, spinning away, full of potential. But potential is not the same as actual exposure. The hazardous situation occurs when your shoelace comes loose and dangles near the chain while you are pedaling. Now, you are exposed to the hazard. The chain has not caught the shoelace yet. You have not fallen. Nothing bad has happened. But the conditions for harm to occur are now in place. That is the hazardous situation.

Why this matters: Risk controls must target the correct point in the sequence. Preventing exposure is different from reducing harm after exposure.

In medical devices, hazardous situations are shaped by the clinical environment, the patient population, the user's training level, and the conditions under which the device is operated. The hazards may be identical across settings; the hazardous situations are not.

This distinction is one of the most commonly confused in medical device risk management — and getting it wrong has serious downstream consequences.

The hazards may be identical. The hazardous situations are not. And the risk analysis must account for both.

Harm

Harm is what actually happens to the person.

Your shoelace catches in the chain. You fall. You break your wrist. That broken wrist is the harm — **the actual physical injury.**

ISO 14971 defines harm as injury or damage to the health of people, or damage to property or the environment.

Harm exists on a spectrum. A mild, temporary skin irritation is harm. Permanent neurological damage is harm. Death is harm. The spectrum matters enormously, and it connects directly to the next concept — severity. But the first step is simply to name the harm correctly and specifically. The harm should be described in terms of what actually happens to the person.

Why this matters: If harm is described vaguely, severity cannot be estimated accurately — and the entire risk evaluation becomes unreliable.

Harm must be described specifically and clinically. "Adverse patient outcome" is not a harm. "Thermal burn," "hypoglycemia," or "loss of therapy" are harms. An organization that describes harm vaguely, like "adverse patient outcome," "device-related injury", cannot estimate severity accurately, cannot set meaningful risk acceptance criteria, and cannot evaluate whether its risk controls are actually protecting the right people from the right outcomes.

The Sequence That Holds It All Together

Hazard → Hazardous situation → Harm.

These three concepts form a sequence — a chain of events that, if uninterrupted, leads from potential to consequence. The hazard is the source of potential harm. The hazardous situation is the circumstances of exposure. The harm is the outcome.

On your bicycle: chain (hazard) → loose shoelace near spinning chain while riding (hazardous situation) → broken wrist from fall (harm).

This chain forms the foundation of ISO 14971. All aspects of risk management — identification, estimation, control, and evaluation — depend on understanding this sequence correctly.

Why this matters: Flattening the sequence (e.g., calling a failure mode a hazard) leads to flawed analyses and misdirected risk controls.

Probability

Once you understand the sequence, the next question is: **how likely is it to play out?**

Probability is the likelihood that the sequence of events — from hazardous situation to harm — actually plays out.

Your shoelace is loose. It is dangling near the chain. How likely is it that the chain actually catches it? That depends on a number of things. How close is the shoelace to the chain? How fast are you pedaling? Are you riding on a smooth road or a bumpy path that might cause more movement? Have you ridden this way before without incident?

Probability is not a feeling, and it is not a guess — though in risk management it is often both of those things in practice, and being honest about uncertainty is part of doing it well. In medical device risk management, probability is estimated using whatever information is available: clinical literature, field complaint data, testing results, knowledge of similar devices, knowledge of the clinical environment. For a new device with no field history, probability estimates carry more uncertainty than for a device with years of post-market surveillance data. That uncertainty is not a reason to skip the estimate — it is information that should be reflected in the analysis and monitored as the device accumulates real-world data.

Two common misconceptions:

1. **Probability of device failure ≠ probability of harm.** A device can fail without causing harm, and harm can occur without a device failure.
2. **Low probability ≠ acceptable risk.** Probability must always be considered with severity.

Why this matters: Probability alone tells you nothing about how much a risk matters.

Severity

Severity is **how bad the harm is** when it occurs.

If your shoelace catches in the chain and you fall, the severity of the harm depends on how you fall, what you land on, how fast you were going, whether you were wearing protective equipment. A scraped palm is low severity — painful, temporary, fully recoverable. A broken collarbone is moderate severity — significant, requiring medical attention, but recoverable. A traumatic head injury is high severity — potentially permanent, potentially life-altering, potentially fatal.

Severity is an attribute of the harm, not of the event that caused it. The same fall, from the same bicycle, at the same speed, can produce harms of very different severity depending on the circumstances of impact. In risk management, severity is assessed at the level of the harm — what is the worst credible outcome of this hazardous situation leading to harm? — and it is assessed independently of probability. The severity of a harm does not change because the harm is unlikely. A low-probability, high-severity harm is still a high-severity harm. The rarity of its occurrence does not reduce the gravity of the outcome when it does occur.

In medical devices, severity is typically characterized on a scale — from negligible or minor at one end, through serious injury, to permanent impairment and death at the other. Different organizations define these levels slightly differently, but the logic is consistent: the scale exists to create a common framework for comparing harms that are qualitatively very different from each other and ensuring that the most severe potential outcomes receive the most rigorous attention.

Why this matters: A rare catastrophic harm is still catastrophic. Rarity does not reduce severity.

Risk

Risk emerges through the **combination of** the concepts of **probability and severity.**

In terms of ISO 14971, these two factors in combination, where "what is the likelihood that a harmful event will occur?" and "how severe would that event be?", represent the concept of risk. Risk cannot be represented by one or the other of these factors; rather, it consists of both combined.

Think about what this means for your bicycle. A very likely harm of very low severity is a low risk, because although it happens fairly regularly, it is minor and recoverable. A very unlikely harm of very high severity is a high risk despite its rarity, because when it occurs the consequences are grave.

This is why risk cannot be assessed one dimension at a time. Risk management requires holding both dimensions simultaneously and making reasoned judgments about their combination.

In practice, most organizations use a risk matrix — a grid that places severity on one axis and probability on the other, dividing the resulting space into zones such as acceptable and unacceptable risk. The specific dimensions of that matrix, and the criteria for each zone, are decisions the manufacturer must make and document. ISO 14971 does not prescribe them, but the expectation is that the company defines them, uses them consistently, and be able to justify their rationale. This demand for an organization to establish its criteria and be judged against them is among the aspects of risk management that move it from being merely technical to being organizational.

Risk Control

Once you understand the risk, the next question is: **what are you going to do about it?**

This is where ISO 14971 prescribes not just that you act, but how you prioritize your actions. There is a hierarchy — and it is not optional or arbitrary. The hierarchy exists because different types of risk controls are fundamentally different in their reliability, and the standard requires manufacturers to always prefer the most reliable option before resorting to less reliable ones:

1. **Inherently safe design** — design out the hazard or exposure
2. **Protective measures** — reduce the likelihood or severity
3. **Information for safety** — warn or instruct

First: design it out. On your bicycle, this is the chain guard — a smooth plastic cover that encloses the chain completely. Now your shoelace cannot reach the chain regardless of whether it comes loose, regardless of whether you remember to tuck it in, regardless of whether you are in a hurry or distracted or simply did not think about it. The hazardous situation cannot occur. The hazard still exists — the chain is still spinning — but the exposure pathway has been closed by the design of the device itself. This is what ISO 14971 calls inherently safe design. It is the gold standard of risk control, because it does not depend on anyone doing anything correctly. It protects every rider, in every circumstance, without requiring knowledge, attention, or correct behavior from the person being protected.

Second: add a protective measure. If the chain cannot be fully enclosed — perhaps the design requires the chain to be exposed for mechanical reasons — then maybe think of a physical guard that deflects a caught shoelace before it can fully engage the chain, reducing the force of the incident even if it cannot prevent it entirely. Or protective equipment — a helmet and knee pads that reduce the severity of the fall if it does happen. These measures still work without requiring the rider to do anything correctly in the moment of exposure. They are engineered into the system. They are less powerful than inherently safe design because they only control the consequences but are far more reliable than the third option.

Third, and only when neither of the first two is feasible: provide information. A warning label on the bicycle, or an instruction in the manual, or a reminder printed near the chain: tuck in loose clothing before riding. This is what ISO 14971 calls information for safety. It is not worthless — a well-designed warning, clearly placed and clearly worded, does address the risk. But it is the weakest form of risk control, because it depends entirely on the rider reading the warning, understanding it, remembering it, and acting on it — every single time, including when they are rushed, distracted, tired, or simply did not notice the label. A chain guard protects every rider, but a warning label protects only the rider who happens to follow it.

Why this matters: This hierarchy — design it out, protect against it, warn about it — is one of the most important ideas in all of medical device risk management. It will appear in almost every chapter of this book, because almost every function makes decisions towards the device risk. Neither of them may think of their work in those terms. But the hierarchy connects them, whether they know it or not.

Residual Risk

After you have applied your risk controls — the chain guard, the helmet, the tucked laces — some risk remains.

Not because you have failed. Because that is the nature of risk in a physical world. The chain guard might be damaged. The helmet might not be worn correctly. A rider might fall in a way that no protective measure could have prevented. Some residual possibility of harm exists no matter how well the risk controls are designed and implemented.

This remaining risk that is left after all possible risk controls have been applied, is called residual risk.

Residual risk is not a failure of risk management. It is the expected output of it. The goal of risk management has never been to eliminate all risk. That goal is not achievable for any device that performs any meaningful function. The goal is to reduce risk as far as possible or reasonably practicably, taking into account the current state of technology, the feasibility of further risk reduction, and the benefit the device provides —

and then making a clear-eyed judgment about whether the risk that remains is acceptable given what the device offers in return.

This is the point where many organizations become uncomfortable, because it requires an explicit acknowledgment: there is no such thing as a zero-risk medical device. Every device on the market carries residual risk.

Why this matters: There is no such thing as a zero-risk medical device. Pretending otherwise prevents honest evaluation.

Benefit-Risk

If risk cannot be reduced to zero, the next question is: **is the remaining risk justified by the benefit?**

The answer is benefit-risk determination — the evaluation of whether the benefits of a device outweigh the risks it carries.

Go back to your bicycle.

A bicycle without any risk is a bicycle that does not move. The moment it moves, there is the possibility of falling. And yet billions of people ride bicycles every day, and the existence of that possibility does not make bicycles unacceptable. Nobody expects a bicycle manufacturer to guarantee that no rider will ever fall. What they expect — what is reasonable to expect — is that the manufacturer has made falling as unlikely and as survivable as possible, and that the residual risk of riding is clearly outweighed by everything that riding offers: freedom, speed, efficiency, joy, physical health, connection to the world.

The benefit justifies the residual risk. Not because the risk is zero. Because the benefit is real, the risk has been reduced as far as possible or is reasonably practicable, and the balance between them is favorable.

That is benefit-risk analysis. And that is, in essence, what ISO 14971 asks of medical device manufacturers.

In medical devices, benefit-risk determination is a clinical judgment informed by evidence, alternatives, and feasibility of further risk reduction.

This is why benefit-risk cannot be assessed in isolation from the clinical purpose of the device. Risk management that considers only the risk side of the equation — treating every residual risk as a problem to be solved without reference to what the device offers — will arrive at conclusions that do not serve patients. Sometimes accepting a risk is the right decision for a patient. Sometimes it is the only decision that gives the patient a meaningful option at all. Risk management done well holds the full picture.

And risk management done honestly acknowledges, clearly and without evasion, what residual risks exist — so that patients, clinicians, and regulators can make informed decisions about whether the benefit justifies them.

Why this matters: Risk management that ignores benefit produces decisions that do not serve patients.

The Lifecycle: Risk Management Does Not Have an End Date

There is one more concept that completes the vocabulary of this chapter, and it is perhaps the most consequential one for how organizations structure their risk management systems.

Risk management is not something you do once.

Your bicycle does not stay the same forever. For example, the chain may stretch with use, or the tires may wear, or the brakes may lose their sensitivity. You may start riding in conditions you did not originally plan for — wet roads, nighttime, steeper hills. None of this was visible when you first assessed the risks of riding. Some of it was foreseeable in principle but not certain in practice. Some of it genuinely could not have been anticipated until it happened.

Medical devices work exactly the same way. The risk assessment produced during device development — even a thorough, rigorous, well-resourced risk assessment — is a snapshot. It reflects the knowledge that existed at the time it was produced, about a device whose real-world behavior in a real patient population had not yet been observed. It is the best analysis possible given what was known. It is not, and cannot be, the final word.

ISO 14971 is explicit on this point: risk management is a lifecycle process. It begins at the earliest stages of device conception and continues through design, development, manufacturing, post-market surveillance, and all the way to device discontinuation and decommissioning. At every stage, new information can emerge that is relevant to the risk picture — field complaints, post-market clinical data, changes to the device or its manufacturing process, new knowledge about the clinical environment, changes in the patient population. All that information has to feed back into the risk management file and be evaluated for its implications.

This means that the risk management file is a living document, not an archive. It is not completed when the device receives regulatory clearance or approval. It is updated — continuously, systematically, for the life of the device — as new information becomes available. An organization that treats design-phase risk management as the end of its risk management obligation has misunderstood the framework at the most fundamental level.

Why this matters: A risk file frozen at design transfer is not a risk file. It is an artifact.

The Vocabulary, Complete

Hazard. Hazardous situation. Harm. Probability. Severity. Risk. Risk control. Residual risk. Benefit-risk. Lifecycle integration.

These are the ten concepts that the rest of this book is built on. Not because they appear in ISO 14971, but because they describe the reality of what risk management is trying to accomplish, which is identifying what can go wrong, understanding how and why, reducing the risk as far as possible, being honest about what remains, and continuing to learn from the device's behavior in the real world for as long as it is in use.

Every chapter that follows will use this vocabulary. Not heavily, not technically, but as the common language that allows a project manager, a manufacturing engineer, a clinical safety specialist, and an executive to talk about the same thing and understand each other.

This chapter gives you that language. The rest of the book will show you how to use it.

Chapter 3: The Total Product Lifecycle – Risk Never Sleeps

A Device Is Never Finished

Every medical device development process has one point where it seems complete to the team. It could be when the design is finally completed, or when approval comes from the relevant authorities. It could also be the day that the first production device leaves the factory floor and arrives at its destination, which could be the hands of the end user. What was once a mere idea, then an experimental prototype, has now become a reality performing its actual function.

It is a significant moment and deserves to be recognized. But it is not the end of risk management.

A medical device enters the real world carrying the critical thinking and risk analysis of the people who designed it — their knowledge, their assumptions, their best estimates of how the device would be used and what could go wrong. No matter how careful and rigorous the analysis was, it was based on information that the real world will eventually correct. Patients use devices in ways that clinical studies might not fully capture. Clinical environments create conditions that laboratory testing might not fully replicate. There may be variability in manufacturing processes that no one foresaw. Failure modes will show up after time that are not identified in accelerated testing.

This is where risk management comes in. It does not occur only once, but throughout the entire product life cycle.

ISO 14971 is very clear about this. Risk management is a lifecycle process. It begins at the earliest moment of device conception, and it does not end until the last unit of that device is decommissioned and out of service. Every phase of the device's life — from the first conversation about what the device should do, through design and development and manufacturing and launch, through years of post-market existence, through design changes over the course and all the way to the end — is a phase in which risk management has a role to play and in which risk-based decisions are being made, whether the people making them know it or not.

This chapter maps that lifecycle at a high-level: what risk management is doing at each phase, what decisions carry patient safety implications at each stage, and how the information generated at every point feed into a continuous, living understanding of whether this device is safe enough for the patients who depend on it.

Concept Design: The Phase Where Risk Management Should Begin — And Rarely Does

The design control process starts with user needs. Before a single engineering requirement is written, before any design input is documented, the development team is asking a foundational question: what does this device need to do, for whom, under what conditions, and in what clinical environment?

These questions are the raw material of risk management.

The intended use of a device — who will use it, how they will use it, where they will use it, what they will use it for — defines the hazard landscape. A device intended for use by trained clinical specialists in a controlled hospital environment carries a different set of hazardous situations than the same device intended for use by patients at home, unsupervised, potentially with limited dexterity or literacy or technical familiarity. The clinical indication determines which patient populations will be exposed to the device, and therefore which harms matter most and at what severity levels. The use environment determines what external factors, for example electromagnetic interference, temperature variation, user fatigue, time pressure, might interact with the device in ways that affect safety.

All of this is known, at least in outline, at the concept stage. And all of it should be informing the earliest risk thinking, even before there is a design to analyze. What hazards are inherent to the clinical domain this device is entering? What does the state of the art in similar devices tell us about where the risks arise? What does the clinical literature tell us about the harms that matter most for this patient population?

Risk management that begins at concept design arrives at the first formal hazard analysis with a foundation of a preliminary understanding of the hazard landscape that makes the analysis completer and more reliable. Risk management that begins only when someone asks for a risk assessment, i.e., after user needs are written, after design inputs are drafted, after the project is already well underway, is starting late. And starting late means the earliest design decisions, the ones with the most leverage over safety, were made without it.

Design Planning: Establishing the Risk Management Framework

Design planning is where the development project gets its structure, like its phases, its gates, its deliverables, its resource plan. It is also where the risk management plan should be established.

The risk management plan is not a risk assessment. It is the framework document that defines how risk management will be conducted for this device, what risk acceptance criteria will be used, what methods will be applied, who is responsible for which activities, and how risk management will integrate with the rest of the design and development process. Getting the risk management plan right at this stage matters because it sets the rules that every subsequent risk decision will be measured against.

Risk acceptance criteria are particularly important to establish early. These are the thresholds that define when a risk is acceptable, when it requires further reduction, and when it is unacceptable regardless of further reduction. They need to be set ***before*** the risk analysis is performed — not after. An organization that defines its risk acceptance criteria after seeing the results of its hazard analysis has created a circular process that cannot be trusted. The criteria exist to evaluate the analysis, not to be shaped by it.

Design planning is also where the scope of the risk management activities is defined, by understanding which standards apply, what related processes need to integrate with risk management, and how design changes will be assessed for their safety impact. The decisions made in design planning create the architecture that the rest of the risk management process inhabits. When that architecture is well-designed and clear, the risk management that follows is more likely to be meaningful. On the other hand, if it is treated as a formality, the risk management that follows tends to be more of a documentation exercise than value-add.

Product Design: Where the Hazard Landscape Takes Shape

As design inputs are established and the design process begins, the device starts to become real in a way that makes a detailed risk analysis possible and necessary. The design inputs — the requirements the device must meet — each carry risk implications. Some requirements exist specifically because of safety considerations: performance limits, material specifications, electrical safety parameters, sterility requirements. Others are functional requirements that, if not met, could create hazardous situations. The risk management process at this stage is mapping the relationship between what the device is required to do and what can go wrong if it fails to do it.

This is the phase where the hazard analysis takes its first substantive form. The design team is making architecture decisions — choices about how the device will be structured, what components it will use, how those components will interact — and each of those decisions shapes the hazard landscape. For example, a design that relies on software to control a safety-critical function carries different risk considerations than a design that implements that function in hardware. These are risk decisions made by engineers who may be thinking primarily about performance and cost and manufacturability — and they need to be made with the risk implications visible.

The design review at this stage is not just a technical milestone. It is a risk management checkpoint. Are the design inputs complete enough to support a meaningful hazard analysis? Are the preliminary risk controls incorporated into the design? Are the highest-risk features of the design receiving the most rigorous engineering attention?

The design phase is also iterative. Designs evolve; requirements evolve; components get substituted; features get added or removed. Any of these actions has the possibility to alter the risk profile – to add new hazards, to change hazardous conditions, to impact the efficacy of risk controls that have already been implemented. Risk assessment during this phase is an ongoing activity that parallels the design process, keeping the risk document current with the evolving design, reflecting the actual product and not just the imagined one.

Design Verification: Testing to the Level of Risk

Design verification determines whether design outputs conform to design inputs — in other words, whether the device performs according to its specifications. It is a core design control activity, but it is also the stage where the connection between testing and risk management becomes most visible. Unfortunately, this is also where that connection is most often overlooked.

Verification must reflect the **risk significance** of the requirement being tested. A safety-critical requirement — one whose failure could lead to a hazardous situation with serious harm — demands more rigorous testing than a requirement whose failure would cause only minor inconvenience. This does not diminish the importance of non-safety-critical requirements; it simply means that verification resources must be allocated proportionally to the safety impact of the requirement.

This is why the verification plan cannot be created independently of the risk management file. The risk analysis identifies which requirements are safety-critical, which failure modes carry the highest risk, and where verification must be most robust. When verification planning and risk management are disconnected, the organization ends up with two documents that do not inform each other — and that disconnect has direct implications for patient safety.

Verification also provides the evidence that **risk controls actually work**. Many risk controls are embedded in the design itself — a hardware interlock, an alarm, a barrier, and a software limit. Verification confirms that these controls are present and effective. If a risk control fails verification — if the interlock does not engage, or the alarm does not trigger at the correct threshold — then the risk control is not functioning, and the associated risk remains uncontrolled. Verification is the moment where that truth becomes visible.

Design Validation: Confirming Safety in the Hands of Real Users

Design validation is more extensive than design verification. Whereas design verification considers whether the design satisfies its specifications, design validation assesses whether the device satisfies the requirements of the intended users and patients. Validation occurs under **conditions similar to those expected** when using the device.

In terms of risk management, design validation can be seen as the stage at which the hazardous scenarios developed during hazard analysis are validated against reality. The clinical setting, users, and conditions of use cease to be abstract concepts during design validation. Instead, these are the real-life factors in which the device will be used by actual users undertaking genuine clinical work.

At this point, use-related risks are highlighted. While a device might be perfect during design verification, it may not perform well when used by nurses in a stressful and chaotic emergency department setting. It is possible for a device to meet all its specifications but still present use error hazards beyond what was considered during hazard analysis. Design validation allows for these flaws to be detected before the product is launched in the market.

The clinical studies and usability evaluations conducted as part of validation activities provide input data to risk management. The results of a summative usability test, in particular, play a direct role in determining whether use-related risks have been adequately managed and the adequacy of the risk controls used to manage them. If a summative test uncovers a critical use error, it informs the risk management process that there is a higher likelihood of the hazardous event occurring than was previously determined in the risk analysis or that there may be a problem with the effectiveness of the risk control.

The final product reviewed in the design validation process forms the basis for the benefit-risk determination. This is where an organization formally and explicitly determines whether the benefits of using the device outweigh its risks. Given what is now known about the device — how it performs, the risks that remain, and its usage by actual users in realistic clinical conditions — should the benefits be considered to exceed the risks?

Design Transfer: Handing Over More Than Drawings

Design transfer is the phase that is most frequently treated as a purely technical handoff — the moment when the device design moves from development to manufacturing, when drawings and specifications and process documentation become the basis for production. Get the documents right, complete the transfer checklist, close the design history file. Done.

It is not done.

Design transfer is a risk management event. The manufacturing processes established during transfer determine how reliably the design — and the risk controls embedded in it — will be reproduced across every unit produced. A risk control that exists in the design but is not faithfully reproduced in manufacturing is not an effective risk control. It is merely a design **intent**. There is a significant difference between the two, and that difference lives in the manufacturing process.

This means that the risk management file needs to be consulted during design transfer to identify which design features are safety-critical, which specifications carry the most risk if they are not consistently met, and which manufacturing processes therefore require the tightest controls. The process validation and production controls established during transfer should be commensurate with the safety significance of what they are controlling. A feature whose out-of-specification condition creates a high-severity hazardous situation requires more robust process controls — tighter tolerances, more frequent monitoring, more sensitive detection methods — than a feature whose variation produces no safety consequence.

Design transfer is also the point at which the risk management responsibilities that lived primarily in development begin to shift toward manufacturing and quality. The people who will produce this device, inspect it, test it, and release it now need to understand which aspects of their work carry patient safety significance. For instance, what are the important aspects, what cannot be changed about the material, what will be dangerous if done wrongly in the assembly process? This knowledge needs to be conveyed intentionally.

Production: Where Risk Controls Either Hold or Fail

Once the device is in production, risk management does not recede into the background. It becomes more operational.

Every manufacturing process is a risk control or supports one. The conditions under which a device is assembled, tested, inspected, packaged, and sterilized determine whether the risk controls embedded in the design are faithfully reproduced in every unit that leaves the facility. Production controls such as the procedures, the inspection criteria, the environmental specifications, the equipment calibration requirements, exist to ensure that consistency. And the rigor of those controls should be proportionate to the safety significance of what they are controlling.

The principle that manufacturing engineers apply instinctively to quality in general is tighter tolerances on more critical features, or more frequent monitoring of higher-risk processes. However, the patient safety dimension of that same principle is not always as visible. For example, a change to a manufacturing work instruction — even a change that seems purely administrative, like reordering steps for efficiency — has the potential to affect the safety of the device produced under it and therefore requires evaluation against the risk management file before it is implemented.

Non-conformances discovered during production are also risk management considerations. A component that fails incoming inspection, a device that fails end-of-line testing, a process that drifts outside its validated parameters — each of these is a data point about the relationship between the manufacturing process and the device's safety characteristics. Some non-conformances will have no safety significance. Some will have significant safety implications that are not immediately obvious. The only way to know the difference is to evaluate them against the risk management file and to ask questions such as whether the failure mode observed in manufacturing is characterized in the hazard analysis, whether it affects a risk control, and whether the risk associated with it needs to be revisited. This is how the risk management system learns from production reality and maintains its relevance to the device actually being manufactured.

Post-Market Surveillance: The Risk Management System Meets the Real World

Once a device is on the market, risk management becomes a real-world activity. Patients and clinicians use the device in diverse environments, under varying conditions, and in ways that no pre-market testing can fully anticipate. All of this use generates information — about performance, failures, use errors, and unexpected interactions with clinical practice.

Post-market surveillance (PMS) is the structured process of collecting, analyzing, and acting on that information. Under ISO 14971, PMS is not optional or passive; it is a continuous obligation to monitor real-world safety and feed what is learned back into the risk management file.

Information arrives through many channels: patient and user complaints, regulatory reports (such as FDA MedWatch and MAUDE submissions or EU MDR vigilance reports), clinical literature, registry data, post-market studies, and observations from service engineers who repair and maintain devices in the field. Each channel is a way for the real world to communicate with the risk management system.

The key question is always the same: **Does this new information change what we know about the device's risks?** Does it reveal a previously unidentified hazard? Does it show that a known risk occurs more frequently than expected? Does it indicate that a risk control is less effective in practice than it appeared during development?

Organizations that treat PMS as a compliance task tend to miss these signals. Organizations that treat PMS as a safety process use this information to update the risk management file, revise probability estimates, reassess risk controls, and — when necessary — reconsider the benefit-risk balance. PMS is how the risk management system stays honest once the device meets the real world.

Corrections, Removals, and Recalls: When the Risk-Benefit Balance Shifts

Sometimes post-market surveillance reveals something that cannot be addressed through a risk re-assessment and a CAPA. Sometimes the information that comes back from the field such as accumulated complaint data, post-market study results, a pattern of adverse events, indicates that the device's benefit-risk balance has shifted in a way **that requires action in the market**.

A field safety corrective action, or a recall, or a correction. These are not admissions of failure in the sense that they are evidence of a broken development process. They are, in many cases, the risk management system working exactly as it should — identifying that the real-world evidence no longer supports the pre-market benefit-risk determination, and taking action to protect patients before the harm accumulates further.

The decision to initiate a correction or removal is itself a risk-based decision. It requires weighing the risk of the device continuing in service against the risk of the corrective action itself (by disrupting use of the device that patients and users are relying on). Additionally, the possibility that removing or modifying the device creates its own safety implications. It requires regulatory engagement and it requires communication — to customers, to clinicians, to patients, to regulators — that is accurate, timely, and sufficient to enable the people in the field to take appropriate action.

The organizations that handle corrections and removals most effectively are the ones that have maintained a living risk management file throughout the device's lifecycle — one that reflects current knowledge, current post-market surveillance findings, and current benefit-risk thinking. When the time to act arrives, they have the analytical foundation to make a well-informed decision. The organizations that struggle are typically the ones for whom the risk management file represents a snapshot from design freeze, never updated, bearing increasingly little relationship to what the device has revealed itself to be in years of real-world use.

End of Life: The Lifecycle Closes, The Obligation Does Not Immediately

A medical device reaches its end of life if the manufacturer decides to discontinue it. It means that the manufacturer stops making the device, withdraws it from the market, and starts developing the next generation of the device. Discontinuing a device can be viewed as a risk management issue, which is not always clear.

When a device is discontinued, it does not mean that the device will no longer be used in clinics. Patients may continue using the device without having any choice. In some clinical categories — implants, therapeutic devices, devices used in rare diseases with few treatment options available — there might still be some devices in use after years of being discontinued.

The risk management issues associated with such devices do not disappear at the moment of discontinuing the device.

Manufacturers remain responsible for all risk management tasks related to the discontinued device, including its post-marketing surveillance, complaint handling, and vigilance reporting. The risk management file still needs to be considered if the device is actively used by patients. Sometimes field corrective actions should be taken, post-market surveillance data should be collected, and benefit-risk assessment should be reconsidered. Discontinuation ends manufacturing, not responsibility.

The end of the device life is where the entire lifecycle of the product, the unbroken curve from conception to development to manufacture to post-market life, completes itself. Risk management insights gained during the lifespan of the product become the basis for the new device. What risks could not be foreseen? Which risk mitigation strategies performed sub-optimally? What new insights emerged from post-market data analysis that should influence the creation of the follow-up product? Not only is this learning that takes place. It is output from the risk management process with patient safety implications that should not be lost in the move from one product generation to another.

The Thread That Runs Through All of It

Throughout this chapter, we followed a medical device from its earliest concept to its final clinical unit. Across every phase, one truth remained constant: **risk management is not a phase, a deliverable, or a milestone. It is a continuous way of thinking.**

Risk management is a thread woven through every decision, every gate, every review, every investigation, and every piece of information that enters the system. It is present whether the people involved recognize it or not. The manufacturing engineer revising a work instruction may not think of herself as influencing the risk management file. The complaint handler closing a field report may not see himself as contributing to a benefit-risk determination. A service technician noticing an anomaly during a repair may not realize he is surfacing a safety signal that the post-market surveillance system needs.

Yet each of these actions is part of the same thread.

Risk management is not a task performed by a department; it is a responsibility carried by an entire organization. It lives in the decisions made by engineers, clinicians, quality specialists, project managers, service teams, and executives. It lives in the questions they ask, the assumptions they challenge, the data they surface, and the choices they make.

The chapters that follow take this thread and make it visible. Each chapter focuses on one function, in one part of the lifecycle, and shows — specifically and concretely — what risk management asks of that function. What decisions carry patient safety implications? What information matters? What responsibilities are unique to that role?

The answers differ for every function. But the thread is the same for all of them.

Chapter 4: Risk-Based Decision-Making Across the Quality System

There is a version of the quality management system that most people in medical device organizations know well. It is the infrastructure of compliance, i.e., the collection of procedures, records, audits, reviews, and corrective actions that regulators expect to see and that auditors come to assess. It has a structure, a documented hierarchy, a set of processes that connect to each other in ways that the organization's quality manual describes. It exists, in the minds of many people who work within it, primarily as the system that keeps the company in good standing with the FDA and the notified bodies.

The quality management system is also the organizational infrastructure through which risk-based decisions are made about a medical device. Every major process in the quality system is a point at which information about the device's safety reaches either to the patient or back to the manufacturer, gets evaluated, and either triggers action or does not. Every one of those evaluations is a risk-based decision. For example, the CAPA that gets opened or closed, the change that gets approved or rejected, the complaint that gets escalated or closed, the management review that identifies a trend or misses one. Each of these moments is the quality system's integration with risk management, and the quality of the decision made at each moment determines how well the organization understands the safety of the devices it puts into the world.

The QMS is not just a compliance framework; it is the organizational machinery through which safety-critical decisions are made every day.

This is the connection that Chapter 3 established from a product lifecycle perspective: risk management is woven into every phase of the device's life. This chapter establishes the same connection from the quality system perspective: risk management is woven into every process of the quality infrastructure. The two pictures together — product lifecycle and quality system overview— give you the complete map of where risk-based decisions live in a medical device organization.

Design controls were the starting point of that map in Chapter 3. They will not be repeated here. If you have read Chapter 3, you already understand how risk management integrates with design inputs, design outputs, verification, validation, and design transfer. What this chapter addresses is what happens in the rest of the quality system — the processes that operate throughout the device's life, and that are equally important to the risk management picture and equally dependent on risk-based thinking.

Production and Supplier Control: Where Risk Controls Either Hold or Erode

The manufacturing floor is where design intent becomes physical reality — where specifications become parts and where assembly procedures become devices.

Process and production control is the quality system element that governs this translation. This includes processes related to the procedures for building devices, the controls associated with ensuring that the devices have been built properly, systems associated with traceability from raw materials to devices, and processes associated with the supplier of quality parts so that when those components arrive at the manufacturing facility, they comply with the design specifications.

In terms of risk management, the central question that underpins all of this is always the same: Is the level of control appropriate based on the safety impact of the controls?

Think about the implications of that statement. Not all manufacturing steps are created equal in terms of their impact on patient safety. Risk-based process control means that the organization has thought explicitly about patient safety and criticality, and has allocated its monitoring, its inspection, its process validation rigor, and its tolerance limits accordingly.

The same logic applies to supplier quality. A supplier who provides a decorative component with cosmetic variation presents a different risk than a supplier who provides a safety-critical component whose dimensional tolerances directly affect device performance in a clinical setting. Supplier qualification requirements, incoming inspection criteria, supplier monitoring frequency, and the response to supplier non-conformances should all reflect that difference. An organization that applies the same oversight to every supplier regardless of the patient safety significance of what they supply is not doing risk-based supplier management. It is doing uniform supplier management — which wastes resources while missing what matters.

The risk management file is the reference point for these decisions. It identifies which design features are safety-critical, which specifications carry the most risk if not consistently met, and therefore which manufacturing and supplier controls need to be most robust. In such cases, where the relationship is established, that is, where those involved in process/supplier control decision making have proper access to the risk management file, the system will consistently work towards patient safety. Otherwise, production control and supplier management turn out to be quality systems operating independently of its purpose, namely, safety analysis.

Change Management: The Risk Decision Nobody Always Recognizes

Change is constant in medical device organizations. Designs evolve, manufacturing processes improve, suppliers change their materials or their facilities, software gets updated, procedures get revised, etc. At any given moment, in any functioning medical device organization, changes are being assessed, approved, implemented, and closed across a dozen different systems and processes.

Every change needs to be assessed for safety risk.

This is not an exaggeration. A change to a device such as its design, its materials, its manufacturing process, its software, its labeling, etc. has the potential to alter the hazard landscape established by the original risk analysis. It may introduce a new hazard, or it may change the conditions under which an existing hazardous situation can occur, or it may affect the effectiveness of a risk control, or it may alter the probability or severity of a harm. Or it may do none of these things. But the only way to know which is true is to evaluate the change against the risk management file with the specific knowledge of what the risk analysis contains and what the change affects.

The challenge is that changes arrive in many forms, and not all of them are immediately recognized as having safety implications. A design change that modifies a structural component in a way that affects load-bearing performance is obviously safety-relevant, and most organizations will recognize it as such. A change to the order of manufacturing steps, made for efficiency, may not trigger the same instinct, and yet if those steps include or precede a safety-critical assembly operation, the change must then be assessed to understand what it means to patient safety as a result. A software update that fixes a display bug may seem cosmetic, and yet if the display communicates safety-critical information to the clinical user, the update touches a risk control.

Change Management, the quality system process that governs how changes are initiated, reviewed, approved, and implemented, is the organizational mechanism for catching these implications before the change is made rather than discovering them afterward. A change assessment process that explicitly asks whether a proposed change affects any hazard, hazardous situation, or risk control identified in the risk management file is a change management process that functions as a patient safety gate. One that asks only whether the change affects form, fit, or function in the absence of any connection to the product risk management file, is a change management process that is systematically blind to the safety implications of the decisions it approves.

Risk review as part of change management is not an additional burden placed on the people who manage changes. Rather, it is the mechanism by which the risk management file stays current with the device as it actually exists, rather than the device as it was designed years earlier. A risk management file that is never updated to reflect changes to the device it governs is a historical document, not a safety tool.

Corrective and Preventive Action: Where the Quality System Learns from Risk

CAPA — corrective and preventive action — is the quality system's learning mechanism. It is the process by which the organization identifies that something has gone wrong, or could go wrong, investigates the root cause, implements a solution, and verifies that the solution has worked. Done well, it is one of the most powerful tools in the quality system.

In terms of risk management, CAPA assumes an important place. CAPA is the only QMS process that explicitly closes the loop between real-world failures and the risk management file. Whenever the occurrence of a non-conformance, the investigation of a customer complaint, or the findings of an audit highlight some aspects regarding the product or production process that were unforeseen during the risk assessment process, CAPA allows bringing that information into the company's attention.

The risk-based dimension of CAPA operates at two levels.

The first is in deciding which issues warrant a CAPA at all. Not every non-conformance, every complaint, or every observation requires a formal CAPA — and organizations that open CAPAs for everything rapidly accumulate a backlog that makes it difficult to focus attention on the issues that actually matter. Risk-based prioritization of CAPA activity means that the decision about whether to open a CAPA, and how urgently to investigate it, is informed by the patient safety significance of the issue as one of the factors. For example, an issue that affects a safety-critical device function, that implicates a characterized hazardous situation, or that recurs in a pattern suggesting a systemic failure, warrant urgent, thorough CAPA investigation. An issue that has no safety consequence and represents an isolated occurrence of a minor procedural deviation warrants a different level of response.

The second level is in the investigation and solution itself. A root cause investigation that reveals a gap in the risk management framework, such as a hazard that was not identified, or a risk control that was not effective, or a probability estimate that was too low, etc. needs to address the risk management file as well as the root cause as a corrective action. A CAPA needs to fix a product issue through an informed risk management process in this scenario.

Product Surveillance: The Quality System's Ear to the Ground

Product surveillance — covering complaint handling, risk monitoring, and vigilance reporting — is the quality system element most directly analogous to the post-market phase described in Chapter 3. It is the set of processes through which information about the device's real-world performance reaches the organization and gets evaluated for its risk implications.

The key difference between good product surveillance and otherwise is not in how much data is gathered but, in the analysis, performed on the data gathered and in how well conclusions drawn are traced back to the risk management record.

Complaint analysis is the primary source of raw material. Any complaint about a device - any communication received from the customer, from the doctor, or from a patient regarding an unexpected, malfunctioning, or problematic event involving the device - could potentially provide information about how the device is behaving in reality with respect to its hazards. There will be some complaints that are due to operator errors and misuse. Some will just be single incident occurrences. Some will be patterns indicating that the risk situation was occurring at a frequency beyond what was originally estimated.

Not only is the issue of reportability an important concern when dealing with individual complaints; there is also the concern over how a particular complaint will affect knowledge regarding the risk profile of the device. For example, an individual complaint may have little effect on the overall risk profile. However, a series of complaints may suggest that a reassessment of the probability dimension of a defined risk is necessary or that a hazardous situation exists that was not previously identified during the risk analysis process.

As part of this Quality System process, risk monitoring is the process of analyzing the total pool of post-market information – complaints, field data, post-market study data, the literature, registry information – and asking that question in a systematic way. Is the medical device operating within the risk profile we established? Are there new risks arising from our information sources that are changing our risk profile? Are there hazardous conditions arising in use that have not been identified by our risk analysis? The key is not just collecting data but making a systematic connection between that data and the risk management file. Neither will do the job alone.

Management Responsibility: The Risk Decisions at the Top

Management responsibility in the quality management system covers two major activities: management review and internal audit. Both are quality system requirements. Both carry risk management significance that is frequently underappreciated.

Management review is the periodic, formal process by which the organization's leadership assesses the performance of the quality management system — reviewing data, identifying trends, making decisions about resources and priorities and improvements. Under both FDA regulations and ISO 13485, management review is a defined requirement with specified inputs. It is also one of the most important forums in the quality system for risk-based decision-making at the organizational level.

The connection to risk management is direct. Management review should include, among its inputs, the outputs of post-market surveillance, the status of the risk management system, the trends in complaint data and CAPA activity, and any significant changes to the risk profile of products in the portfolio. The decisions that emerge from management review — about where to invest in product improvement, about which quality issues require escalated attention, about whether the organization has the resources and competencies its risk management obligations require — are risk decisions made at the highest level of the organization.

The internal audit is the process by which the quality system checks itself to see if the processes that have been set up are doing their job. The auditors check if processes are being followed, if there are records to prove this, if the quality system is upholding the standards that it is supposed to. In the realm of risk management, the internal audit has a particular importance. It is one of the few ways in which the organization can check itself to see if the risk management system is doing its job.

An internal auditor who understands risk management can evaluate whether the risk management file is being updated to reflect post-market information, whether change assessments are genuinely considering safety implications, whether CAPA investigations are addressing root causes that implicate patient safety, and whether the connections between the quality system's various processes and the risk management framework are functioning as the organization's procedures describe.

The Quality Systems as a Risk Management System

The processes described in this chapter are not risk management processes in a narrow sense. They are quality system processes. But at every decision point, each of these systems ask questions that have patient safety implications: Is this change safe to make? Is this non-conformance connected to a characterized hazardous situation? Is the organization's leadership making resource decisions that reflect the patient safety significance of what they are deciding?

Every one of those questions is a risk-based question. All responses are risk assessments. The effectiveness of these risk assessments – their level of analysis, the correctness of its correlation with the content of the risk management document, the degree of strictness in its implementation – will define, overall, whether the quality management system serves as a patient safety system or as a compliance management system.

The difference between these two concepts cannot be seen in the paperwork. Both will generate records. Both will pass audits, at least most of the time. The difference becomes apparent in terms of patient outcome – in the ways in which harm is avoided through catching the signal, evaluating its impact correctly, solving a CAPA and controlling product risk, as well as making the right resource management decision.

That is what risk-based decision-making across the quality system means. Not a different set of processes. The same processes operated with the risk management file as a genuine reference point rather than a parallel document that the quality system acknowledges without consulting.

A QMS that does not integrate risk is a compliance system; a QMS that does integrate risk is a safety system.

The Logic of ISO 14971

Before diving into the functional chapters, it helps to understand the simple logic that sits underneath every clause of ISO 14971.

The reasoning is based on a simple principle, proven in Chapter 2: all medical devices have some risk associated with them. No medical device that produces any effect, whether it is the transfer of energy, the transmission of a substance, the supply of information for clinical decision making, or the replacement or support of physiological processes, is risk-free; risks associated with them cannot be eliminated but must be understood and mitigated to an acceptable degree.

ISO 14971 is the standard that formalizes this process. Its logic is straightforward: identify hazards, estimate and evaluate the risks they create, determine which risks are acceptable, reduce the unacceptable ones, evaluate the residual risk against the device's clinical benefits, and continue monitoring the device throughout its life. Every clause in the standard is simply a specification of one part of that sequence.

That is it. That is the whole framework. Every clause in ISO 14971 is a specification of one part of that logic, i.e., what it means to identify hazards systematically, how risk estimation should be approached, what constitutes a valid risk control, how benefit-risk should be evaluated, what the post-market monitoring obligation looks like. The standard is detailed because each of those steps has enough complexity to warrant specificity. But the underlying logic is simple enough to state in a brief paragraph, and by keeping this logic in view makes it much easier to understand why each requirement exists. And ISO/TR 24971 provides the detailed guidance that supports this logic, expanding on the concepts and offering practical interpretation.

However, here is the **honest reality:** the majority of people in a medical device organization will never read ISO 14971. That includes many of the people whose daily decisions have the most direct impact on whether the risk management framework is functioning as it should.

The project manager who decides when the risk assessment needs to be completed is making a decision that ISO 14971 has something to say about. Risk assessments require complete inputs, and development timelines must account for that dependency. The project manager does not need to have read ISO 14971 to understand that. But someone needs to have translated it.

The manufacturing engineer who assesses a change to a work instruction is making a decision that ISO 14971 has something to say about — changes to production processes must be evaluated for their risk management implications. The engineer does not need to be fluent in the standard, but they need to understand the principle behind the requirement: that a change to how the device is built has the potential to affect the risk controls built into the design, and that potential needs to be evaluated before the change is implemented.

And that is the translation issue that this book aims to address. ISO 14971 was drafted for risk managers who have sufficient technical expertise to translate its guidance directly into a tangible device-related application. But the other members of the organization require the essence of the guidance, translated into terms that relate to their world. And that translation is what the chapters in Parts II–V of this book do.

ISO 14971 gives you the guidance. This book gives you what that guidance means for you. Your function. Your decisions. Your role in the grand scheme of the risk management framework.

Part II— Design & Development Functions

Chapter 5: Marketing & Product Management

Ask a product manager whether their work touches product risk management and the answer is often a confident yes — usually followed by a description of attending design reviews, reviewing risk assessments, and signing off on design inputs. Ask whether their work directly shapes the safety profile of the device, and the answer becomes more hesitant.

In most organizations, the story goes like this: Marketing and Product Management define what the device needs to do and who it needs to serve, then hand that definition to engineering, which builds the device. Risk management is seen as everything that happens **after** this handoff — something that lives in engineering, in quality, or in the risk file created during design and verification.

This leaves a critical gap.

The intended use statement — what the device does, how and by whom, where it is used, and under what circumstances — is not a marketing artifact. It is the foundational input to the entire risk management process. Every hazard identified, every hazardous situation analyzed, every risk control designed and verified, every benefit-risk determination made — all of it traces back to the intended use. Change the intended use, and you change the hazard landscape. Expand the user population, and you change the foreseeable use errors. Add a clinical indication, and you may introduce hazardous situations nobody has analyzed. Narrow the intended use for regulatory convenience, and you may create a gap between how the device is evaluated and how it is actually used.

The person who writes the intended use statement is making decisions that directly shape product risk. In most organizations, that person works in Marketing or Product Management — and in most organizations, nobody has told them that.

This chapter is that conversation.

What Marketing and Product Management Actually Own

Before discussing where the risk decisions live, it helps to clarify what Marketing and Product Management actually do — because the function varies across organizations. In some companies, Marketing owns voice-of-customer research, intended use development, and product claims. In others, Product Management owns product requirements and the development roadmap while Marketing handles commercial strategy and promotion. In many organizations, the two functions blend depending on the stage of the product lifecycle.

For this chapter, what matters is the set of decisions and outputs this combined function produces — because those outputs carry patient safety significance.

These outputs fall into two broad categories:

1. **Defining what the device is** — intended use, intended users, clinical environment, performance claims, indications.
2. **Communicating what the device is** — promotional materials, sales messaging, clinical education, field communication.

The first shapes the risk analysis from the inside. The second can distort or expand the safety profile externally in ways the risk management file may never see.

The Intended Use Statement: More Than a Sentence

The most consequential output Marketing produces — and the one that shapes the entire risk analysis — is the intended use statement.

The intended use describes the device's clinical purpose, identifies the patient population, and specifies the setting in which it is meant to be used. It is often drafted early and then treated as a fixed reference point.

ISO 14971 requires manufacturers to begin risk management by characterizing the intended use and the population of patients who will be exposed to the device. The intended use is not just context for the risk analysis. It is the input that makes the analysis possible. Without a clearly and accurately defined intended use, the hazard identification process has no boundary — and therefore no reliable way to determine whether it is complete.

Consider what the intended use actually specifies, and what each element means for risk:

1 Who will use the device

This determines the use-error landscape. A device intended for trained specialists carries different foreseeable use errors than one used by general practitioners or patients at home. If the intended user population is defined too narrowly, the use-error analysis will miss scenarios the real-world user population will encounter.

2 Who the patient population is

This determines which harms matter most and at what severity. A device used on pediatric patients carries different severity implications than the same device used on healthy adults. A device used on patients with multiple comorbidities, or on patients who are already in a compromised physiological state, sets a different risk landscape than a device used on low-risk patients undergoing elective procedures. The patient population is not just a commercial characterization. It is a safety characterization.

3 Where the device will be used

This determines the environmental hazards and the conditions under which the device must operate reliably. A device intended for use in a controlled hospital environment operates in a different use environment than a device intended for pre-hospital emergency use, or home use, or use in low-resource settings. The noise levels, the lighting, the availability of support personnel, the likelihood of interruption, the power supply reliability — all of these are environmental factors that shape the hazardous situations the device can create or encounter.

4 What the device is intended to do

This determines the inherent hazards — the energy, the substances, the mechanical forces, the information outputs that are intrinsic to the device's function. For example, a device that delivers a drug carries the hazard of incorrect dose delivery, a device that provides diagnostic information carries the hazard of incorrect information influencing a clinical decision, and so on. The intended purpose is the starting point for hazard identification, and the accuracy with which it is defined determines how complete that identification can be.

Each of these elements is typically defined by Marketing or Product Management — often early in development and under commercial pressure, without the explicit understanding that these are risk decisions with downstream consequences throughout the device's lifecycle.

Why this matters: Every hazard analysis, risk control, and benefit-risk decision depends on the intended use being accurate.

Reasonably Foreseeable Misuse: The Risk Nobody Wants to Name

Intended use defines the ideal scenario. Reasonably foreseeable misuse defines the real one.

ISO 14971 requires manufacturers to consider not only hazards arising from intended use but also hazards arising from reasonably foreseeable misuse — the ways in which users might interact with the device outside its intended purpose, predictably, based on what is known about how users behave in clinical practice.

This is not reckless or negligent misuse. It is predictable misuse based on:

- clinical context

- device design
- known patterns of use for similar devices

For example, a device that is designed for single use but that clinicians routinely attempt to reuse in cost-constrained settings is subjected to reasonably foreseeable misuse. A device that is approved for one patient population but that clinicians regularly apply to an adjacent population with similar presentations is being used in a way that is reasonably foreseeable even if not intended.

Marketing and Product Management have visibility into this reality that no other function has. They talk to clinicians. They attend clinical conferences. They hear from sales teams who observe real-world use. They see the gap — often early — between intended use and actual use.

That visibility is valuable. When this information reaches the risk management file, the hazard analysis reflects clinical reality. When it stays within commercial conversations, the risk file describes a device being used as intended in a world where it is not.

The question is not whether Marketing knows about off-label use or uses outside the intended patient population. In most organizations with commercially active products, they do. The question is whether that knowledge has a structured path into the risk management file and understanding that responsibility in the product's safety risk management process.

Why this matters: Devices fail in the gap between intended use and actual use.

Voice of Customer as Safety Data

If intended use defines the boundaries of risk, voice of customer reveals the terrain inside those boundaries.

New product development begins with understanding what the market needs. Marketing and Product Management lead clinician interviews, field observations, surveys, and competitive analysis. These activities shape design requirements — and they also shape the hazard landscape.

User needs that accurately reflect how clinicians will actually use the device — what tasks they will perform, in what sequence, under what conditions, with what level of attention and training — enable a hazard analysis that captures the real use-error landscape.

It is at the stage of translation of voice of customer to design inputs for development that the hazard landscape is set. In effect, if a clinical observation pointing to a potential safety issue — say a clinician observes that the display is difficult to interpret in certain lighting conditions, and so on — is excluded from consideration during the derivation of user needs, the hazardous situation doesn't go away, it just remains untreated.

Marketing and Product Management do not need to perform hazard analysis themselves. But they must ensure that safety-relevant observations reach the risk management file. VoC is a powerful risk management tool — but only if treated as safety data, not just commercial input.

Why this matters: Early-stage clinical insights are often the first signals of future hazardous situations.

Promotional Claims and the Gap Between Promise and Evidence

Marketing claims are not just commercial statements. They shape clinical decision-making.

A manufacturer's claims about a particular medical device, whether presented in promotional material, in clinical studies, or during the process of selling the medical device, are not mere marketing information. These claims relate to the capacity of the medical device and what can be expected from it when it is used on patients. If these claims are accurate, the clinician will make informed decisions about what should be done. However, when the claims exaggerate what the device can do, then another risk has been introduced into the equation.

A clinician deciding which devices to use will make a decision that is influenced by the claims made. If the claim is true and is backed by evidence, then the decision is an informed one. However, when the claim goes beyond what has been studied about the device and what can reasonably be expected of it in various conditions, then the decision may not be based on evidence and the facts about the medical device itself.

This is not only a regulatory compliance concern but also a patient safety concern. The gap between what a promotional claim implies and what the device has actually been demonstrated to do is a gap in the benefit-risk evaluation. The benefit that justifies the device's residual risks is the benefit that has been clinically demonstrated, not the benefit that is implied in a marketing brochure.

Marketing and Product Management typically develop and approve promotional materials. That responsibility includes ensuring claims are accurate, evidence-based, and consistent with the evaluated intended use.

Why this matters: A claim that overstates benefit distorts the benefit-risk balance clinicians rely on.

Promotional Materials as an Unrecognized Surveillance Source

Information flows both ways — and the reverse flow is often ignored.

Organizations understand the outward flow: clinical data, promotional claims, labeling, training materials. What is less understood is the inward flow: observations, questions, unexpected behaviors, and real-world use patterns that return through commercial channels.

Sales teams hear it. Medical science liaisons hear it. Training sessions reveal it. Clinical education events surface it. Key opinion leaders articulate it.

In the vast majority of companies, none of this information has an organized channel to get into post-market surveillance processes or the risk management database. It gets into the sales process, into sales meetings, into the relationship management process. Some of it influences the development of the next set of promotional materials, but very little of it ever finds its way into the complaint handling process, post-market surveillance database, or the risk management process.

This is a systemic issue — and only Marketing and Product Management can fix it, because they control the channels through which this information flows.

A product manager who understands their post-market surveillance obligation builds a structured process for capturing and routing safety-relevant information — and understands why it belongs in the risk management system, not just in commercial discussions.

Why this matters: Commercial channels are often the earliest source of post-market safety signals.

The Risk-Based Decisions You Make Every Day Without Knowing It

For a product manager or marketing professional, risk-based decisions appear in everyday work:

- **When you write or approve an intended use statement**, you decide which hazards the risk analysis will examine — and which it will not.
- **When you define the intended user population**, you determine which use-error scenarios human factors must address.
- **When you identify a new market opportunity**, you may be observing evidence of off-label use that requires risk evaluation.
- **When you approve a promotional claim**, you make a statement about what the device can safely and reliably do.

- **When you capture voice-of-customer feedback,** you are receiving post-market surveillance data — and you play a critical role in ensuring it reaches the risk management file.

These decisions happen in strategy meetings, customer conversations, and the daily work of sustaining a commercial product. They are risk decisions nonetheless — and patients depend on the people making them to understand that.

What Risk Management Actually Needs from You

I hope this chapter has made clear how Marketing and Product Management contribute to the device's risk management process — and the risk-based decisions embedded in their daily work.

To sum it up, risk management needs you to understand that the intended use statement is the most consequential risk document in the entire product file because everything that follows from it in the risk management process depends on its accuracy and completeness.

It needs you to recognize that the clinical information flowing into your organization through commercial channels is post-market surveillance data that needs to flow into the risk management file to re-evaluate safety claims of the device.

It needs you to understand that a new indication, a new market, a new user population, or a new clinical setting is a risk management event before it is a commercial event — and that the risk analysis needs to precede the promotion, not follow it.

And it needs you to bring the same rigor to the clinical accuracy of your promotional claims that you bring to their commercial effectiveness – because the claim that reaches a clinician is the information on which a patient care decision will be made, and the patient at the end of that decision is depending on the claim being true.

You define what the device is for. You define who it is for and where it will be used. You communicate what it can do.

All of that is risk management — and you play a critical role in it.

Notes & Sources

- **On user needs and design inputs** — ISO 13485:2016, Clause 7.3.3.
- **On post-market surveillance and the obligation to collect and review field information** — ISO 14971:2019, Clause 10; ISO/TR 24971:2020.

Chapter 6: Program & Project Management

Project and program managers in medical device organizations are, in a very practical sense, the people most responsible for whether risk management actually happens — and the people least often described that way.

Ask a PM whether they own product risk management, and the answer is usually no. They own the schedule, the budget, the plan, and the "project risks," but nothing related to the device. They facilitate the cross-functional team, manage gate reviews, and drive decisions that keep the project moving. Risk management is what quality does. It is what happens in the risk file. It has its own team, its own procedure, and its own deliverables that appear on the project plan as milestones to be checked off.

This is a reasonable description of how most organizations are structured. It is not a complete description of how safety decisions actually get made.

Because the decisions that determine whether risk management is genuine — whether design inputs are complete, whether safety findings are addressed before a gate or pushed into the backlog, whether a design change is evaluated for safety implications — all happen in the PM's domain. They happen in project planning meetings, in scope reviews, in resource allocation discussions, and in the gate reviews the PM prepares and drives. They happen when a PM looks at a design change assessment form and decides who needs to review it.

This chapter is not a critique of PMs. It is an argument that nobody has explained to them which of their daily decisions affect patient safety — and what asking the right question actually looks like. A PM who understands this is not just a better PM. They are a genuine patient safety asset in a role where the organization desperately needs one.

What Program and Project Managers Actually Do

Before mapping where risk lives in PM work, it helps to be honest about the scope of what PMs actually manage — because it is broader than most people outside the role appreciate.

A project manager in medical device development is the cross-functional integrator. They hold together the activities of engineering, quality, regulatory, clinical, manufacturing, marketing, and suppliers — all working on different parts of the same problem, with different priorities, timelines, and definitions of done. The PM is the one person who sees all of these pieces simultaneously and recognizes when something happening in one discipline has implications for another.

That visibility is extraordinary. It is also why the PM's understanding of safety risk management is consequential.

Program managers carry an even broader view. They manage portfolios of projects, oversee the strategic product roadmap, and make resource allocation decisions across multiple development programs. Their risk-relevant decisions operate at a higher level: which programs with safety implications need priority; which safety findings from one project should be shared across the portfolio; which design platforms carry known safety limitations that every new project must account for.

Both roles sit at the center of a network of choices that determine patient safety.

The Full Map: Every Place Risk Lives in a PM's Work

Project planning and scheduling

When risk management activities are scheduled as deliverables with due dates — "risk assessment complete by March 15" — rather than as processes with prerequisites, the schedule is structurally set up to produce a document rather than an analysis.

Risk assessment needs finalized intended use. Hazard analysis needs a sufficiently defined design. Risk control verification needs a stable design and test methods derived from the risk analysis.

These are not arbitrary preferences. They are dependencies. If compressed or reordered under timeline pressure, the risk analysis becomes less capable of doing what it exists to do.

Why this matters: A risk assessment done with incomplete inputs is not a risk assessment — it is paperwork.

Resource allocation

Risk management takes time. Thorough hazard analysis, meaningful cross-functional review, and careful evaluation of risk controls cannot be accelerated without degrading quality.

If a PM allocates three days to assess a complex design change, the risk manager has three days. Whether that is enough depends on the device, the modification, and the available information. And the output of the assessment may itself require additional design work, additional verification, or additional risk controls.

This is an iterative analysis throughout the project. A PM who understands this allocates time based on complexity and safety significance — not on what fits neatly into the Gantt chart.

Why this matters: Under-resourced risk management leads to under-analyzed risk.

Gate and milestone management

Phase-gate reviews are one of the most important safety mechanisms in development.

A gate review that asks, "Is the risk assessment complete?" is asking whether a document is signed. A gate review that asks, "Was the risk assessment performed with the inputs available at this stage, and are those inputs sufficient for meaningful analysis?" is asking whether the organization actually knows what it needs to know before proceeding.

Why this matters: Gate reviews are safety checkpoints — not administrative ones.

Design change management — where the most visible failures happen

Design changes are the most concentrated intersection of project management and patient safety — and the most common place where the gap between the two becomes consequential.

Every design change — to a requirement, component, software module, manufacturing process, material, or configuration — has the potential to affect the device's risk profile.

Some changes are obviously safety-relevant: for example, a modification to the algorithm controlling a therapy delivery function, or a substitution of a structural component with different load-bearing characteristics, etc. Others are less obviously connected to safety: for example, an internal software refactoring that does not change any visible function but still affect risk controls or hazardous situations.

The PM's role is not to perform the safety assessment. It is to ensure:

- the assessment happens
- the right people perform it
- the risk file is consulted
- the conclusion is based on actual analysis

The gap occurs when someone informally concludes "no safety impact" without reviewing the risk file. The change moves forward. The risk file remains unchanged. And the device in the field no longer matches the device described in the safety analysis.

The PM who catches this gap needs only one question: "What in the risk file was reviewed to support this conclusion?"

Why this matters: Most post-market safety issues trace back to design changes that were never evaluated for safety impact.

Scope management

Scope creep is a project risk. In medical device development, it is also a patient safety risk when the additions to scope are not evaluated for their safety implications.

A new feature added during development is, from a risk perspective, a design change. It may introduce new hazards, interact with existing risk controls, or alter use scenarios.

A PM who manages scope with a risk lens is not blocking innovation. They are ensuring that every addition is evaluated for safety before it becomes part of the device patients will encounter.

Why this matters: Every new feature is a new risk scenario until proven otherwise.

Escalation and communication

When the risk management team raises a concern — a hazard that cannot be controlled, a risk control that failed verification, a safety finding requiring design change — the PM's response determines what happens next.

A PM who escalates safety concerns ensures leadership makes conscious risk acceptance decisions. A PM who asks for a workaround to protect the timeline is making a risk acceptance decision they are not authorized to make.

Escalating safety findings is not the same as stopping projects. It is ensuring that the people who are responsible for making risk acceptance decisions such as leadership, appropriate clinical or medical authority, etc. have the information they need to make those decisions consciously rather than by default.

Why this matters: Silence is an implicit risk acceptance — and PMs have the ability to escalate safety concerns.

Two Kinds of Risk Management — and Why PMs Need to Know the Difference

PMs are trained to manage risk. But project risk and product safety risk are not the same.

- **Project risk** affects the project — schedule, budget, scope, resources.
- **Product safety risk** affects the patient — hazards, hazardous situations, risk controls, harm.

A schedule delay is a project risk. A software module that fails to control a hazardous situation is a product safety risk.

A project risk register and a product hazard analysis are not interchangeable. Both are necessary. Both must be done. But neither replaces the other.

Why this matters: Confusing project risk with product safety risk is one of the most consequential errors in medical device development.

Software Changes, Agile Development, and the PM's Unique Challenge

Software-intensive development introduces a tension earlier generations of device development did not face.

Waterfall development mapped reasonably well to design controls: requirements → design → verification → validation. Risk management could be scheduled around these phases.

Agile development does not work that way. Features evolve in sprints. Design decisions are incremental. Software changes rapidly and continuously, and the change between each sprint may not be formally characterized as a design change in the traditional sense.

This creates a real challenge: The risk management process must stay current with what the software actually does — and agile development can outpace traditional risk assessment cycles. A hazard analysis performed at the beginning of development may no longer accurately describe the software after six sprints of iterative feature development.

AAMI TIR45 addresses this tension. It provides guidance on integrating risk management into agile rhythms rather than treating it as a separate activity between sprints.

For PMs, the key takeaway is simple:

Risk management must be built into the sprint rhythm.

During each sprint review, the PM should ask:

- Did anything change that affects a safety-critical function?
- Did any risk control change?
- Did any hazardous situation change?
- Do the new features introduce new risk?
- Has the risk analysis been updated accordingly?

Why this matters: If the software changes and the risk file does not, the organization loses control of safety.

The Questions Every PM Should Be Asking

These are not technical questions. They are judgment questions — and they make the difference between genuine safety risk management and the appearance of it.

- **At project initiation:** Does the project plan give risk management enough time with the right inputs?
- **At every gate review:** What was the risk management team able to analyze at this stage, and what could they not yet analyze because the design was not sufficiently defined? What safety questions are still open, and what is the plan for answering them?
- **For every design change:** What in the risk file was reviewed to support the conclusion?

- **For every scope addition:** Does this introduce a new hazard or affect existing risk controls?
- **When a safety concern is raised:** Who needs to know, and what decision must they make?
- **In every agile sprint:** Did anything change in this sprint that is connected to a safety-critical function, a risk control, or a characterized hazardous situation? If yes, have the right risk management activities been performed before the sprint is closed?
- **For resource allocation:** Is the time allocated to risk management proportionate to the safety significance and complexity?

None of these require expertise in ISO 14971. They require understanding that PM decisions shape the environment in which risk management happens — and the quality of that environment determines whether the risk management system can do its job.

What Risk Management Actually Needs from You

Risk management needs PMs to understand that the schedule, gates, resources, and change assessments they drive are not separate from safety. They are the conditions under which safety analysis succeeds or fails. It requires PMs to:

- Build risk checkpoints into sprint reviews, design reviews, phase gates, and scope decisions.
- Recognize that product safety risk does not appear in the Gantt chart — it appears in the field months later.
- Use their influence to ensure safety questions are asked at the right time.

You have more reach into the risk management system — and more ability to influence how the organization approaches safety — than any job description acknowledges. Use it.

Notes & Sources

- **On the distinction between product safety risk management and project risk management** — ISO 14971:2019; ISO 31000:2018.
- **On design and development planning and gate management** — ISO 13485:2016, Clause 7.3.2.
- **On agile development and medical device software risk management** — AAMI TIR45:2012/(R)2018, *Guidance on the use of agile practices in the development of medical device software.*
- **On design change control and risk management implications** — ISO 14971:2019, Clause 10.2; ISO 13485:2016, Clause 7.3.9.

Chapter 7: Systems Engineering & Architecture

Systems engineers in medical device organizations are, in a very specific sense, one of the closest technical functions to the risk management process. They understand failure modes, redundancy, fault tolerance, and system-level reliability. They think in sequences of events and consequence chains. They draw architecture diagrams that show exactly what happens when a component fails and how the system responds.

The architecture decisions made early in development — long before the design is stable enough for formal analysis — determine which hazards can occur, which hazardous situations are possible, and which risk controls are even available to the teams that follow. Everything downstream — every hazard analysis, every risk control specification, every verification test — operates within the design space that systems engineering created.

That is an extraordinary amount of patient-safety leverage. This chapter makes that leverage visible — and focuses on the concepts that are most consequential and most frequently missed.

The Architecture Is the First Risk Control

Architecture decisions are safety decisions inherently — whether or not they are labeled that way.

Before a single formal risk analysis is performed, the system architecture has already made a set of patient-safety decisions. It determines:

- Which functions are centralized or distributed — and therefore where single points of failure may exist.
- How the device responds to failure modes, such as sensor failures, power interruptions, software faults, and communication losses, etc. — and therefore which hazardous situations are possible or designed out entirely.

- Which functions are implemented in hardware and which in software — and therefore what classes of risk controls are available.
- Whether safety-critical functions are isolated from non-safety-critical ones — and therefore how failures can propagate.

These are not aesthetic engineering choices. They are inherently safe-by-design decisions — the top tier of the risk-control hierarchy described in Chapter 2. ISO 14971's hierarchy exists for a reason: inherently safe design is always preferred over protective measures, which are always preferred over information for safety. A system that cannot enter a hazardous state because the architecture makes that state unreachable is safer than a system that can enter the hazardous state but relies on a protective measure or a warning label.

Systems engineers make these hierarchy-defining decisions at the whiteboard, months before the risk management file formally characterizes the hazards they are addressing. The question that should guide these decisions — but is rarely articulated — is: **For each hazardous situation we have identified, does the architecture reduce the possibility of that situation, or must we manage it another way?**

This question does not slow down architecture work. It sharpens it. It gives architectural decisions a safety evaluation criterion and produces an architecture that the risk management file can analyze and leverage — because the safety thinking is already built into the structure.

Why this matters: The architecture determines which hazards are even possible. It is the first and most powerful risk control the device will ever have.

Essential Performance: The Risk-Based Definition That Shapes Everything

Once the architecture defines the system's safety boundaries, the next major risk-based decision is defining essential performance.

Essential performance is formalized in IEC 60601-1 for medical electrical equipment, but the concept applies to any device performing a clinical function. Essential performance is the set of performance characteristics whose absence or degradation leads to unacceptable risk — the functions the device must continue to perform, or must cease performing in a defined safe state, to protect patients from harm.

This distinction matters because devices have many performance requirements — accuracy, speed, display resolution, battery life, communication capability — but only some have safety consequences when they fail. Here's a concrete example:

For an infusion pump:

- **Performance requirement:** The display must refresh every second.
- **Essential performance requirement:** The pump must not deliver more than the programmed infusion rate.

If the display refreshes slowly, the device is annoying. On the other hand, if the pump over-infuses medication, the device is harmful.

Essential performance classification drives:

- Which functions require redundancy
- Which require fault detection and safe-state logic
- Which require environmental and fault-condition testing
- Which require electromagnetic compatibility testing
- Which require reliability targets derived from risk analysis

A systems engineer defining essential performance is making a risk-based determination that requires explicit engagement with the hazard analysis:

- What hazardous situation occurs if this function fails?
- What is the severity of harm?
- What reliability and fault protection does this function require?

If essential performance is defined by competitive benchmarking, customer requests, or regulatory precedent alone, the classification may be technically defensible but functionally unsafe.

Why this matters: Misclassifying essential performance leads to misallocated risk controls — and unsafe devices.

Reliability Determination: Where Risk Acceptance and Engineering Commitment Must Connect

Architecture and essential performance define what must be safe. Reliability determines how consistently it stays safe.

Systems engineers set reliability targets and allocate reliability thresholds across subsystems. They model failure rates and evaluate whether the architecture can meet its reliability goals. This is rigorous, quantitative engineering work.

What is less often rigorous is the connection between reliability targets and risk-acceptance criteria.

In a properly integrated process, the probability of harm estimated in the hazard analysis and the failure rates committed to in the reliability architecture must align. If the hazard analysis concludes that a hazardous situation must occur with a probability no greater than 1 in 100,000 uses, then the reliability target for the function whose failure leads to that hazardous situation must support that probability.

If the reliability target is looser, the risk acceptance criterion is no longer supported by engineering commitment. The residual risk the risk file determines "acceptable" is not the residual risk the device will actually produce.

In practice, this gap is common and largely invisible. Reliability engineers work with tolerance stack-ups and subsystem models. Risk managers work with probability estimates and harm severity. The systems engineer is the only person with the technical breadth to see both sides and close the gap.

Why this matters: A risk acceptance criterion is meaningless if the reliability target cannot support it.

Traceability: The Engineering Discipline That Makes Risk Management Defensible

Once architecture and reliability commitments are set, the next question is: can we prove it?

Traceability is often treated as a documentation obligation — links among requirements, design outputs, and test results for audit purposes. But for risk management, one traceability path matters most:

Hazard → Hazardous Situation → Risk Control → Design Output → Verification → Evidence of Effectiveness

When this chain is intact, the risk documentation describes a coherent safety story. When any link is missing — for example, a design output that does not trace back to a risk control, or a verification test that does not trace back to the hazardous situation it was intended to control — the organization cannot demonstrate that the device is safe.

Example of traceability done well

- Hazard: Over-infusion
- Hazardous situation: Pump delivers fluid faster than programmed
- Risk control: Software interlock limiting maximum flow rate
- Design output: Flow-rate limiting algorithm

- Verification: Test confirming algorithm limits flow under fault conditions
- Effectiveness evidence: Simulation showing clinicians can respond in time

Example of traceability done poorly

- Hazard identified
- Risk control listed
- Verification test exists
- But no link between the test and the hazardous situation
- No evidence the control actually interrupts the hazard sequence

The systems engineer holds the key to this architectural relationship. If the architecture is done well, traceability emerges naturally. If not, traceability becomes an after-the-fact reconstruction — incomplete, fragile, and misleading.

The actual result of this failure of traceability is more than just vulnerability to regulatory action. The failure means that the company cannot answer the critical question: Given our understanding of this hazardous situation, what evidence can we produce that shows that our risk control measure actually reduces the risk? If the answer requires manually searching through disconnected documents to reconstruct a connection that should have been maintained throughout development, the answer is probably incomplete — and the risk file's residual risk conclusions are based on evidence the organization cannot fully justify.

Why this matters: Without traceability, the organization cannot prove that its risk controls work — and cannot defend its residual-risk conclusions.

Verification of Implementation Versus Verification of Effectiveness: The Distinction That Most V&V Programs Miss

This is the most frequently missed distinction in systems engineering's relationship to risk management, and the one with the most direct patient safety consequences.

ISO 14971 requires two separate verifications for every risk control:

1. **Verification of implementation** — confirming the control is present in the device.
2. **Verification of effectiveness** — confirming the control actually reduces the risk.

Most organizations perform the first. Few perform the second.

3. **Implementation verification asks:**
    - Is the interlock present?
    - Is the alarm threshold set correctly?
    - Is the guard installed?

These questions can be answered by examining design outputs.

4. **Effectiveness verification asks:**
    - Does the interlock prevent the hazard under fault conditions?
    - Does the alarm activate in time for a clinician to respond in the real environment?
    - Does the guard prevent exposure under foreseeable misuse?

For example, an output that confirms an alarm activates at 120 milliliters per hour is verification of implementation. A test that confirms the alarm activates at 120 milliliters per hour and that clinical users in a realistic simulation of ICU conditions actually notice and respond to it within a clinically meaningful time window is a test of effectiveness — because it connects the control to the hazard sequence it was designed to interrupt, not just to the specification it was designed to meet.

The difference is profound. Effectiveness testing requires knowledge of the hazardous situation — the sequence of events leading from hazard to harm. That knowledge lives in the hazard analysis.

If V&V is designed without reference to the risk file, the tests cannot generate evidence of effectiveness.

Systems engineers are uniquely positioned to close this gap. They sit at the intersection of requirements (what the control must do) and tests (how its performance is confirmed). A systems engineer who understands this distinction can design V&V programs that include risk-based sample-size selection and at least one test that exercises the hazardous situation the control was designed to interrupt.

Why this matters: A risk control that is implemented but not effective is not a risk control.

What the Regulations Are Actually Looking For

Regulatory bodies across major markets share a universal principle: manufacturers must provide objective evidence that hazards have been identified, risk controls have been implemented, and those controls are effective.

United States (FDA QMSR)

FDA's QMSR (which incorporates ISO 13485:2016 by reference) requires traceability from design inputs to design outputs and verification and validation. Design verification must show that design outputs satisfy design inputs — and for safety-critical features, design inputs include risk-control specifications derived from the hazard analysis.

A verification effort that confirms performance specifications but does not confirm risk-control effectiveness satisfies procedural requirements but fails safety requirements.

European Union (MDR 2017/745)

Annex I of the Medical Device Regulation contains the General Safety and Performance Requirements (GSPRs). These require manufacturers to:

- Reduce risks as far as possible through design
- Use protective measures only when design cannot eliminate the risk
- Use information for safety only when protective measures cannot fully control the risk

Evidence of conformity must trace back to the risk management file.

Other markets

Health Canada, Australia's TGA, and Japan's PMDA all require the same fundamental connection:

Hazard → Risk Control → Evidence of Effectiveness

Systems engineers build this connection through architecture decisions, risk-control specifications, traceability frameworks, and V&V design.

Why this matters: Regulators do not want documents. They want evidence that the device is safe — and systems engineering produces that evidence.

What Risk Management Actually Needs from You

Risk management needs systems engineers to understand that:

- The architecture diagram is a major risk-management input.
- Essential performance must be defined explicitly against the hazard analysis.
- Reliability requirements for safety-critical functions must align with risk-acceptance criteria.

- Traceability must connect hazards to evidence — not just requirements to tests.
- V&V programs must include risk-based test plans and at least one effectiveness test for every safety-critical control.

You have more analytical capability than almost anyone else on the development team. The risk management process needs that capability aimed directly at the questions above.

When that happens, the devices that reach patients are not just compliant — they are genuinely safer.

Notes & Sources

- **On essential performance and its risk management implications** — IEC 60601-1:2005+AMD1:2012+AMD2:2020, *Medical electrical equipment — Part 1: General requirements for basic safety and essential performance.*
- **On verification of implementation and verification of effectiveness as distinct requirements** — ISO 14971:2019; ISO/TR 24971:2020.
- **On EU MDR General Safety and Performance Requirements and their design implications** — EU MDR 2017/745, Annex I; ISO 14971:2019.

Chapter 8: Hardware R&D and Electrical Engineering

In medical device organizations, IEC 60601-1 occupies a peculiar position. It is one of the most technically demanding standards in the entire development program — generating hundreds of engineering requirements, shaping circuit design from the first schematic, and influencing insulation strategies, material selections, and layout constraints.

The misunderstanding between hardware engineering and product risk management is not about the technical requirements of the standard. Hardware and electrical engineers typically know IEC 60601-1 in considerable depth. The misunderstanding is about what the standard does — and does not — accomplish in terms of patient safety.

IEC 60601-1 establishes minimum requirements for a defined set of electrical hazards: electrical shock, excessive temperature, fire, mechanical hazards arising from construction, and the failure behaviors of programmable electrical systems. When a device is tested and found compliant, it has demonstrated that it meets those minimum requirements for those defined hazards. That is not a small achievement — it represents rigorous engineering and meaningful patient protection.

But it is not the same as completing ISO 14971 risk management. IEC 60601-1 makes this explicit: It states that the absence of a hazard in the standard does not imply acceptability. A complete risk analysis must identify *all* hazards and determine whether additional controls are required. The standard establishes the floor. Product safety risk management determines whether the device's specific hazard landscape requires anything above that floor — and what evidence demonstrates that the controls are adequate.

Hardware and electrical engineers are closest to that hazard landscape. They understand how the device behaves electrically, how it can fail, what happens to patients and operators under fault conditions, and which design decisions create or control hazardous situations. That knowledge is exactly what ISO 14971 requires for hazard identification — and it does not automatically flow into the risk file unless engineers understand that it should.

This chapter closes that gap: identifying the specific ways in which hardware and electrical engineering decisions *are* patient-safety decisions, and where the risk file depends on this function in ways that are not always made explicit.

Applied Part Classification: The Risk Decision That Sets Everything Downstream

One of the earliest structured decisions in any IEC 60601-1 compliance program is applied part classification. Engineers are fluent in the categories:

- **Type B** — minimal patient contact, most permissive leakage limits
- **Type BF** — direct electrical contact with the patient, tighter limits
- **Type CF** — direct cardiac application, most stringent limits

What is less recognized is that this classification is not merely regulatory. It is a risk-scenario classification: a statement about patient vulnerability to electrical injury.

Example: How classification matters

A CF applied part — such as a pacemaker lead or intracardiac catheter — delivers current directly to the heart muscle, bypassing the body's natural impedance. Ventricular fibrillation can occur at extremely low currents, imperceptible at the skin surface. Combined with real-world power-supply variability in clinical environments, this creates a particularly critical risk scenario.

Applied part classification affects the risk management process because it determines:

- which hazardous situations must be analyzed
- which harms must be characterized

- which isolation and protective measures must be verified

If applied parts are classified without reference to the risk file, the hazard analysis will miss the injury scenarios associated with patient exposure.

The engineer doing applied parts classification lays down the ground rules for evaluating the risk level of the device's electrical hazards. This information should be included in the risk management file at once.

Why this matters: Applied part classification determines the severity of electrical injury and drives the entire leakage-current safety strategy.

Single-Fault Condition Analysis: Hazard Analysis in Disguise

Single-fault condition analysis is one of the most practical risk-analysis techniques in medical device engineering — and one of the most misunderstood. It is often treated as a compliance exercise, when in fact it is the core idea of hazard identification and risk estimation.

IEC 60601-1 defines a single fault as the failure of one protective measure or the occurrence of one abnormal condition. The device must remain free of unacceptable risk under any single fault throughout its lifetime.

Viewed through an ISO 14971 lens, single-fault analysis asks:

- What single faults can occur in this device?
- What hazardous situations do they create?
- What is the probability of each fault?
- What is the severity of the resulting harm?
- Which design features — isolation barriers, protective impedances, fuses, safe-state logic — prevent unacceptable harm?

For example: A simple single-fault scenario

- Fault: A fuse fails open.
- Hazardous situation: Loss of power to a safety-critical function.
- Harm: Therapy interruption.
- Risk control: Redundant power path or safe-state transition.
- Verification: Single-fault test confirming safe behavior.

When engineers perform single-fault testing solely for compliance, they are still performing risk analysis — but the outputs may never reach the risk management file. The failure modes, hazardous situations, and verified controls remain in the 60601 test report instead of informing the ISO 14971 hazard analysis.

The hardware engineer's contribution is not performing a separate analysis. It is ensuring that the outputs of single-fault testing flow into the risk file in the language of ISO 14971.

This is a traceability decision that hardware engineers are positioned to make. It requires understanding that the test protocol and the risk file are describing the same things from different angles — and that the risk management process is only complete when those descriptions are connected.

Why this matters: Single-fault analysis is hazard identification in disguise — and must feed the risk file.

EMC As a Risk Management Activity, Not Just a Certification Milestone

Electromagnetic compatibility (EMC) is another area where compliance and risk management are often treated as separate activities. IEC 60601-1-2 Edition 4 changed that. It explicitly integrates ISO 14971 and requires manufacturers to:

- identify essential performance
- characterize the intended electromagnetic environment
- identify EMC-related hazardous situations
- design immunity requirements based on risk
- verify that essential performance is maintained under foreseeable disturbances

These are risk assessment considerations. They necessitate a complete understanding of the hazard profile of the medical device – more precisely, the identification of functional failures resulting in harm to patients – before developing the EMC verification process. They demand coordination with the risk management team to ensure consistency between the identification of essential performance and the hazard analysis conducted. They demand the design of a test process by which each immunity verification test addresses the corresponding hazardous scenario.

An EMC test plan is therefore not a checklist of standardized tests. It is a risk-based verification program **for that device and its intended use**. The first thing that needs to be established is which of the functions are critical performance functions, failure or degradation of which creates unacceptable risk. The second thing that needs to be established is what kind of electromagnetic interference would this device experience in the environment where it is going to operate. For example,

- A home-use device exposed to a microwave oven

- A hospital device exposed to surgical diathermy equipment
- A wearable exposed to a smartphone transmitting at maximum power

Standard immunity levels represent *minimum* requirements. If foreseeable disturbances in the intended use environment of the device exceed those levels, the risk file must document the scenario — and the device must be tested accordingly.

This is a higher analytical bar than compliance testing alone requires. It is also what ISO 14971 and IEC 60601-1-2 together require. Hardware engineers who understand this framing design EMC verification programs that generate true evidence of safety.

Why this matters: EMC failures often manifest as silent, intermittent, or environment-dependent hazards — and only risk-based EMC testing can detect them.

Alarm System Design Is Risk Control Design

Alarm systems in medical electrical equipment are governed by IEC 60601-1-8. The standard defines alarm priority, signal characteristics, persistence, acknowledgment behavior, and networked alarm behavior.

From a risk-management perspective, every element of IEC 60601-1-8 is a risk-control specification. Alarms are protective measures triggered by hazardous situations the design cannot eliminate. Their purpose is to alert the clinical user in time to prevent harm. In situations where the alert does not go off, the risk control measure has failed to work.

This is not merely a hypothetical problem. Clinical professionals have been shown to develop alarm fatigue to the point of not reacting properly when the device gives off alarms; regulators and other agencies have taken note and recognize alarm fatigue as a contributing factor in adverse situations.

Implications for hardware engineers

- Alarm limits are risk-related values and must be set with the hazard analysis.
- Alarm priority must reflect the severity and urgency of the hazardous situation.
- Verification and validation must demonstrate that alarms are perceivable and actionable in the real use environment — not just audible in an anechoic chamber.

AAMI TIR66 provides guidance on physiologic data and waveform databases for validating alarm algorithms — a resource that directly supports risk-based alarm design.

Why this matters: An alarm that activates but cannot be perceived or acted upon is not a risk control.

What Risk Management Actually Needs from You

Risk management needs hardware and electrical engineers to understand that IEC 60601-1 compliance is the *starting point* of electrical safety, not the end. The standard establishes minimum requirements. The risk-management process determines whether the device's specific hazard landscape requires anything beyond that minimum.

Specifically, risk management needs:

- **Applied part classification** to be reflected in the hazard analysis.
- **Single-fault condition outputs** to flow into the risk management file as hazard-analysis inputs.
- **EMC verification** to be designed as a risk-based activity tied to essential performance and intended environments.

- **Alarm system design** to trace back to the hazards the alarms are intended to control.
- **Ongoing linkage** between electrical engineering decisions and the risk file throughout development and post-market.

Compliance documentation and risk-management documentation are not two different processes. They are two views of the same safety case. Both need to be analyzed, and each is incomplete without the other.

When hardware engineers understand this connection, the devices that reach patients are not just compliant — they are genuinely safer.

Notes & Sources

- **On the relationship between IEC 60601-1 compliance and ISO 14971 risk management** — IEC 60601-1:2005+AMD1:2012+AMD2:2020; ISO 14971:2019.
- **On applied part classification and its risk management implications** — IEC 60601-1:2005+AMD1:2012+AMD2:2020; ANSI/AAMI ES60601-1 (US-adopted version).

Chapter 9: Software Development

Software engineers in medical device companies make risk-management decisions every day — with each sprint, commit, bug triage, SOUP update, and architectural change. In most organizations, they make these decisions without realizing it.

This reflects a deeper structural issue. Under ISO 14971 at the system level and IEC 62304 at the software lifecycle level, software development activities must be considered in risk management. Yet software engineers often focus on the technical requirements of IEC 62304 and do not explicitly consider which of their decisions affect patient safety.

The result is an industry-wide pattern: risk management is seen as something the quality department does *after* the software is built, not as questions developers must ask *while* building it. The risk file reflects how the software was intended to behave. But, the software itself has been shaped by hundreds of daily decisions — classification choices, SOUP selections, anomaly triage, change implementations — all with safety consequences that were never explicitly considered.

This chapter maps those decisions. It is written for software developers who know IEC 62304 technically, but who may not yet see how their everyday work translates into patient-safety language.

Software Safety Classification: A Living Risk Decision

Software safety classification under IEC 62304 is one of the first formal risk decisions in any software development program — and one of the most misunderstood. It is often treated as a one-time determination rather than a living risk judgment that must be revisited throughout the product's lifecycle.

IEC 62304 defines three safety classes for software items, based on the potential harm if the software fails or malfunctions, evaluated before risk control measures within the software itself are applied:

- **Class A** — software cannot contribute to a hazardous situation
- **Class B** — software can contribute to a hazardous situation resulting in non-serious injury
- **Class C** — software can contribute to a hazardous situation resulting in serious injury or death

Classification itself is a risk analysis. It asks: if this software item fails — produces incorrect output, crashes, freezes, or behaves unexpectedly — what is the worst hazardous situation that could result, and what is the severity of harm?

This question cannot be resolved by considering the intended purpose of the software alone. Rather, it needs to be resolved through an analysis of the chain of events starting from the failure of the software through the clinical environment to the patient.

There are two important things to note regarding this approach:

1. Mitigations inside the software do not reduce the safety class.

A Class C module does not become Class B because the developer added an error-detection routine. Classification is based on *pre-mitigation* harm.

2. Classification must be revisited when functionality changes.

A module classified as Class A early in development may become Class B or C if new functionality creates a safety dependency.

For example: A display module originally used only for non-critical information becomes safety-critical when a new feature creates a data dependency between the display and a therapy-delivery function. The classification must change accordingly.

A developer who adds functionality without asking whether it changes the safety classification has made an uninformed decision — and the rigor of verification, documentation, and change control may no longer be appropriate.

Why this matters: Classification determines the rigor of development, verification, and change control. When classification is wrong, everything built on top of it is wrong.

SOUP Management: Daily Risk Work, not a Documentation Exercise

Software of Unknown Provenance (SOUP) includes any software not developed specifically for the device or lacking adequate development records. This could include operating systems, open-source libraries, networking stacks, third-party signal processing components, cloud service APIs, database engines, and any other pre-existing software incorporated into the device's software system.

Software of Unknown Provenance — SOUP — is the IEC 62304 term for any software component that was not developed specifically for the medical device being built, or for which adequate development records are not available.

In most programs, SOUP is treated as a documentation task: list the components, note versions, and file anomaly lists. But SOUP management is actually a risk-assessment activity.

Every SOUP component is a potential source of failure whose causes are outside the manufacturer's control. The manufacturer did not write the code and cannot fully know its failure modes. SOUP management therefore asks:

- What does this component do?
- What happens if it fails?
- Could that failure contribute to a hazardous situation?
- How must those risks be controlled?

For example: A JSON parser library crashes when it receives malformed input. In controlled test environment, there may not be a malformed input, But, in clinical use, a networked device may receive corrupted packets. And the library crash could freeze a safety-critical display or interrupt therapy.

Characterization of the SOUP component is not a one-time process but rather an iterative approach. Vendors of SOUP components maintain lists of their anomaly reports, which are periodically updated based on newly identified flaws, and the manufacturer needs to assess whether these flaws could result in a hazardous situation for the device. According to IEC 62304, manufacturers need to evaluate anomaly reports released by the software vendor for each of the SOUP components.

The correct question is not "Do we use this code path?" but **"Could clinical use trigger this code path?"**

This requires understanding:

- the hazardous situations in the risk file
- the clinical environment
- how real-world conditions interact with the SOUP component

Why this matters: SOUP failures originate outside your codebase — and outside your control. They must be evaluated through a clinical-risk lens, not a functional one.

The Probability Problem Unique to Software

ISO 14971 defines risk as the combination of probability and severity. For hardware, probability can be estimated using reliability data, fatigue curves, and environmental testing.

Software does not behave this way. Software failures are deterministic. If a bug exists, it will manifest whenever the triggering conditions occur. There is no wear-out curve, no statistical distribution of failure times.

This creates a challenge: **How do you estimate probability for software hazards?** IEC/TR 80002-1 addresses this directly. It reframes the probability question:

Not: "How often will the software fail?" **But:** "How likely is it that the sequence of events leading to a hazardous situation will occur in clinical use?"

Thus, the probability assessment moves away from the software failure that can never be estimated precisely enough and focuses on the clinical circumstances under which the said software failure can become a potential hazard — which would most probably happen frequently due to its context.

For example: A race condition occurs only when two sensors send data simultaneously within a 2-millisecond window. In testing, this never happens. In clinical use, a patient movement or environmental disturbance may create exactly that timing.

Probability is therefore based on:

- clinical workflow
- user behavior
- environmental conditions
- device interactions

Documenting this reasoning — which clinical conditions are required, how often they occur, and what controls exist — is the developer's contribution to probability estimation.

IEC 62304 reinforces this by treating software classification as a worst-case analysis: the safety class is determined by the worst potential harm if the software fails, without regard to how likely the failure is. This is appropriate at the classification stage because the rigor of the development process should be calibrated to the severity of the potential harm, not to a probability estimate that may be unreliable. But the probability analysis becomes important when characterizing residual risk.

A developer who knows the difference can make a far more substantive contribution to product safety. The substantive contribution is an actual analysis of what constitutes the trigger, what hazard scenario might result from it, whether this trigger is or isn't likely in the clinical setting, and how to manage the risk in question.

Why this matters: Software failures are deterministic. The probability lies in the clinical context, not in the code.

Anomaly Triage: Every Bug Is a Risk Question Before It Is a Quality Question

Software development always involves anomalies. IEC 62304 does not require defect-free software. It requires that every anomaly be evaluated for safety impact.

IEC 62304 establishes the problem resolution process: 1. anomalies must be evaluated for their impact on safety, and that 2. evaluation must be documented.

Stage 1: Technical assessment

- What is the bug?
- Where is it?
- What causes it?
- What is the functional impact?

Stage 2: Safety assessment

- Could this anomaly contribute to a hazardous situation?
- Does it affect a safety-classified software item?
- Does it involve a risk control (e.g., error detection, alarm logic, safe-state transition)?
- Could clinical conditions trigger the bug?

For example: A UI freeze may seem cosmetic. But if the UI displays dosage information or alarm messages, the freeze could delay clinical response — making it a safety issue.

Also, the documentation requirement for non-actions is often underappreciated. If an anomaly is determined to be non-safety-critical, the rationale must be recorded. Otherwise, auditors cannot distinguish between evaluated anomalies and ignored ones.

Why this matters: A bug dismissed without safety evaluation is a silent risk acceptance — and developers are the first line of defense.

Change Control: The Developer's Position in the Risk Evaluation Chain

Every software change — from a one-line fix to a major refactor — modifies a system that has already been assessed for hazards and risk controls. Some changes are safety-neutral. Some are not.

Developers are uniquely positioned to understand the true impact of a change:

- Does it affect a safety-classified item?
- Does it modify a risk control?
- Does it change timing, threading, or data flow?
- Does it alter a SOUP component's behavior?
- Does it introduce new code paths?

For example: A developer reorganizes a threading model to improve performance. The change alters the timing of a safety-critical loop that checks alarm thresholds. The functional behavior appears unchanged, but the safety behavior is not.

This is why developers must actively participate in change impact assessments because of the depth of their knowledge. A change impact assessment completed by someone who did not write the code and does not understand its internal relationships will miss the implications that only the developer can see.

This does not mean developers should complete the formal risk assessment unilaterally — the formal evaluation involves the cross-functional risk management team and must be connected to the hazard analysis and the risk management file. But it means developers must actively participate in the change impact assessment rather than treating it as a quality process that happens after they implement the change.

Why this matters: Most software-related recalls trace back to unassessed changes.

Agile Development and the Integration of Risk Management

All the concepts above apply regardless of development methodology. Agile introduces additional operational considerations because working software changes every sprint. Development rests on iteration cycles, ongoing delivery of functional code, and flexibility with regard to shifting requirements.

The regulatory requirements surrounding medical device software were formulated based on a process model where planning comes before requirements, which comes before design, which then comes before verification. Incorporating risk management into a process model that deliberately disrupts this sequencing demands clear planning and focus.

AAMI TIR45:2023 provides guidance on integrating risk management into agile development. Its core message is simple: agile development is not incompatible with regulatory requirements and risk management obligations. The regulatory requirements do not mandate a specific development methodology. They mandate that specific activities occur and specific evidence be generated. TIR45 shows how those activities and evidence can be integrated into an agile development rhythm without abandoning either the agility or the safety discipline.

1. The sprint as a risk-management unit

At sprint planning:

- Do backlog items modify safety-classified software?
- Do they affect risk controls?
- Do they involve SOUP with known anomalies?

At sprint close:

- Have safety-relevant activities been documented?
- Have anomalies been evaluated for safety?
- Have changes been assessed for impact on the risk file?

2. Definition of done as a safety checkpoint

A user story is not "done" until:

- safety implications are evaluated
- anomalies are triaged
- changes affecting safety are assessed
- documentation is updated

3. Incremental verification

IEC 62304 requires verification of software items. In agile, verification can occur within or immediately after the sprint. What cannot be deferred is integration of verification evidence into the overall risk management file — the connection between what was verified and the risk control it demonstrates effectiveness for.

4. Backlog grooming as hazard identification

Backlog grooming is an opportunity to ask:

- Does this feature introduce a new hazard?

- Does it modify a risk control?
- Does it require reclassification?

5. Sprint reviews as mini design reviews

Involving quality and regulatory teams ensures safety considerations remain visible throughout development.

6. Continuous risk-file maintenance

Perhaps the most important operational difference between agile and traditional risk management is the frequency with which the risk file must be updated.

In a traditional sequential model, major risk file updates are associated with phase gates. In an agile model, where working software changes every sprint, the risk file must be updated continuously to reflect the actual state of the software. A risk file that is accurate at sprint one and not updated through sprint twenty describes a device that no longer exists.

Why this matters: If the code changes every sprint, the risk file must change every sprint. When they diverge, safety assurance disappears.

What Risk Management Actually Needs from You

Risk management needs software developers to understand that:

- **Safety classification is a living risk decision**, not a one-time label.
- **Anomaly evaluation must begin with a safety question**, not just a technical one.
- **Probability analysis must be based on clinical context**, not software behavior alone.
- **Change control requires developer insight**, because only developers understand the true impact of code changes.

- **Agile development requires risk management to be part of the sprint cadence**, not a separate activity performed after the fact.

The risk management file and the codebase must describe the same device. When they say the same thing, the device is safe. When they diverge, the gap between them is where patients are at risk.

Notes & Sources

- **On IEC 62304 as the medical device software lifecycle standard** — IEC 62304:2006+AMD1:2015, *Medical device software — Software life cycle processes.*
- **On IEC/TR 80002-1 as the bridge between ISO 14971 and IEC 62304** — IEC/TR 80002-1:2009 (AAMI/IEC TIR80002-1:2009), *Medical device software — Part 1: Guidance on the application of ISO 14971 to medical device software.*
- **On agile development and medical device software risk management** — AAMI TIR45:2023, *Guidance on the use of agile practices in the development of medical device software.*
- **On FDA regulatory expectations for software documentation** — FDA, *Content of Premarket Submissions for Device Software Functions* (June 2023).
- **On FDA cybersecurity expectations** — FDA, *Cybersecurity in Medical Devices: Quality System Considerations and Content of Premarket Submissions* (September 2023).
- **On EU MDR expectations for software** — EU MDR 2017/745, Annex I (GSPR).

Chapter 10: Human Factors & Usability Engineering

Human factors engineering is the discipline that turned *"user error"* into *"use error"* — and that shift changed the entire safety landscape of medical devices. Twenty years ago, use errors were routinely dismissed as a failure of the individual clinician or patient. Today, the industry recognizes that devices can be designed in ways that make errors predictable and preventable, and that manufacturers bear responsibility for those design decisions.

This progress is real and significant.

The gap however, is that in most organizations, human factors engineering is treated as a process that runs parallel to risk management rather than as a process **embedded** within it. The usability engineering file (UEF) and the risk management file (RMF) are explicitly treated as separate documents that reference each other — the UEF citing the hazard analysis, the RMF citing summative evaluation results — rather than as two outputs of the same analytical system.

When HF and risk management operate in parallel, each can be completed in isolation without strengthening the other. A risk file may describe use-related hazardous situations that the usability process never evaluates. A usability file may validate tasks that the risk file never identified as hazardous situations. A summative evaluation may pass every metric and still leave unvalidated risk controls for high-severity hazards.

These gaps are rarely obvious. The documents look complete. Procedures are followed. Submissions are defensible. And yet somewhere in the clinical field, a device is in use with a hazard that was analyzed but never controlled — or a risk control that was documented but never verified as effective.

This chapter explains the relationship between usability engineering and risk management — specifically, how each depends on the other in ways most practitioners have never been taught to see. It is organized around the two directions of that relationship: what human factors contributes to risk management, and what risk management contributes to human factors. At every step, the question is the same: What does this activity mean for product **risk** and patient **safety**? How does it interact with the risk file? What **risk-based decisions** must the human factors engineer make?

Before the Handshake: Establishing the Scope Boundary

To understand how HF and risk management interact, we must first define their scope boundaries.

IEC 62366-1 governs *normal use*: the full range of interactions between intended users and the device, including correct use and use errors. Use errors — actions or omissions that produce unintended outcomes — are the domain of usability engineering. They arise from mismatches between device design and user capabilities, expectations, or context. These errors can often be addressed through design: improved interfaces, clearer labeling, better feedback, or more intuitive controls.

ISO 14971 has a broader mandate. It requires manufacturers to address not only use errors but all *reasonably foreseeable misuse*, including *abnormal use*. Abnormal use occurs when users intentionally misuse the product in ways the manufacturer could reasonably foresee.

Examples of abnormal use

- Clinicians continuing to use a device past its functional life because replacements are unavailable
- Patients reusing a single-use device
- Users bypassing safety features because they slow down workflow

IEC 62366-1 cannot address abnormal use through design alone. ISO 14971 must address it through hazard characterization, risk estimation, and evaluation of available controls. As a result, when a human factors engineer completes their process and considers use-related risk management finished, they may have left a category of foreseeable hazardous situations unaddressed.

Off-label use sits in this same space. When a device is used in populations or settings outside its labeled indication, the use scenarios may differ substantially from those characterized in usability engineering. **Off-label use** may introduce:

- new use errors
- new clinical contexts
- new abnormal use patterns

If off-label use is reasonably foreseeable, it must be characterized in the risk assessment — even if it cannot be addressed through usability engineering. If it is frequent or severe enough, it may signal the need to evaluate intended-use expansion or contraindication.

Bi-Directional Handshake between HF and Risk Management

For use-related hazards (i.e., hazards that arise from the interaction between the user and the device), completeness depends on the accuracy of the *use specification* — the intended users, environments, and use flow defined by human factors engineering.

Risk-based decisions in defining the use specification are defining:

- Who are the *real* users in clinical practice — not just the ideal or primary users?
- What environments — including non-ideal ones — will the device actually be used in?
- What use scenarios capture the full range of foreseeable interactions?

Human factors engineers define the use flow. When they define it narrowly to manage the scope of usability testing, they are simultaneously constraining the scope of the hazard analysis.

Why this matters: A use specification optimized for regulatory simplicity rather than clinical reality produces a hazard analysis that is systematically incomplete.

Use-Related Risk Analysis and the uFMEA: Building the Hazardous Situation Database

Once the use specification is defined, the next step is building the use-related hazard library. The use-related risk analysis (URRA) and use-FMEA (uFMEA) are the primary tools through which HF contributes hazards characterizations to the risk file. Their structure maps directly onto ISO 14971 framework by identifying:

- use task
- potential use error
- hazardous situation
- sequence of events
- severity of harm
- risk controls

The task analysis that feeds the URRA — the systematic decomposition of every user interaction with the device into discrete steps — is therefore a hazard identification methodology in ISO 14971 terms. Every task step is a potential use error. Every use error is a potential cause of a hazardous situation.

Risk-based decisions in task analysis

1. Does the analysis include both physical and knowledge tasks? FDA's 2024 URRA guidance formalizes knowledge tasks as required. Examples include interpreting a clinical parameter, or recognizing when device output requires action, or understanding a trend arrow or alarm message.

A device whose knowledge-task hazards are not characterized has a structural gap.

2. Does the analysis reflect each user group? An easy task for an expert may be hazardous for a novice. A task routine for a nurse may be performed differently by a home user.

3. Does the analysis incorporate post-market information from similar devices? Complaint data, MAUDE reports, and literature reviews reveal known use-related hazards that task analysis alone may miss.

Why this matters: The completeness of the task analysis determines the completeness of the use-related hazard library.

Critical Task Identification: The Intersection Where HF Drives Validation Scope

Critical tasks are tasks that, if performed incorrectly or not performed at all, could cause serious harm. Identifying them is one of the most consequential risk-based decisions in usability engineering because it determines the scope of the human factors validation study.

The risk file is the authoritative input. A task is critical because the hazardous situation it leads to has high severity. And that severity analysis is made in the hazard analysis.

This means critical task identification cannot be completed by the human factor engineers alone. It requires reviewing the risk management file — specifically, looking at every use-related scenario and tracing it back to the use task it arose from. Human factors engineer who identifies critical tasks based on intuition or user observation alone, without reference to the risk file's severity characterizations, may correctly identify many critical tasks — but may also miss tasks whose criticality is not obvious from observation but is clear from the hazard analysis.

For example: A task that appears simple — such as confirming a dosage setting — may be critical if an incorrect confirmation leads to serious harm.

Risk-based decisions at this stage include:

- Is every high-severity use-related hazardous situation traceable to a critical task?
- Is every critical task traceable to a characterized hazardous situation?

If a hazardous situation has no corresponding critical task, the validation study will not test the scenario — and the risk control will not be verified.

Why this matters: Critical tasks determine what the validation study actually tests, and the criticality of tasks is identified from the risk management file.

Risk Control Selection: The Hierarchy Applied to Use-Related Hazards

When a use-related hazardous situation requires risk reduction, the risk-control hierarchy applies exactly as it does for any other hazard:

1. **Inherent safe design**
2. **Protective measures**
3. **Information for safety**

For HF engineers, this hierarchy has a specific implication: labeling is always the weakest control. It works only if users read, understand, remember, and act correctly under real-world conditions.

The risk-based decision at this step is that: for each use-related hazard that requires risk reduction, has the manufacturer applied the risk control hierarchy appropriately?

This is where HF engineers and risk management professionals need to work together: the human factors engineer brings knowledge of what design interventions are feasible at the user interface level, and the risk management professional brings the formal evaluation of whether each proposed control is at the highest level of the hierarchy.

When this conversation does not happen, i.e., when risk controls are selected by the human factors team without risk management input, or by the risk management team without human factors input, the resulting controls are often implemented in ways that are not actually effective.

For example,

- Weak control: "Do not insert cartridge upside-down."
- Strong control: A keyed connector that makes incorrect insertion impossible.

Why this matters: Labeling is the most common — and most overused — risk control for use-related hazards.

Residual Risk Evaluation: The Output the Whole Process Is Building Toward

Summative evaluation is not just a study report. It is the **verification of effectiveness** for use-related risk controls.

If summative evaluation shows that representative users can perform all critical tasks without critical use errors, the evidence supports the conclusion that use-related risk controls are effective.

If critical use errors occur, the risk control has failed its effectiveness verification. The risk management process must then respond with:

- redesign
- additional protective measures
- or, as a last resort, information for safety

The cycle repeats until residual risk is acceptable or the benefit-risk determination justifies proceeding.

This is the moment where the bidirectional handshake is most visible: the risk management file identifies a risk control for a use hazard → the usability engineering process verified whether that control worked → and the result of that verification determines whether the residual risk evaluation is acceptable or must be revised.

The two processes are iterative partners, each informing the other until the answer is clear.

Why this matters: Summative validation is the only evidence that use-related risk controls work in real hands.

Post-Market: The Feedback Loop That Closes the Handshake

The handshake between HF and risk management does not end upon marketing of the device. If anything, it intensifies after launch.

Complaints, adverse events, and service data reveal what happens when real users interact with the device in real environments. They may expose:

- use errors predicted pre-market
- use errors not predicted
- scenarios not characterized in the hazard analysis
- risk controls that fail under real-world conditions

AAMI TIR50 establishes that this post-market feedback loop belongs to HF. HF engineers have the tools to interpret complaint data through a use-error lens.

Example: A pattern of complaints shows users consistently misinterpreting a symbol. The summative study did not reveal this because the simulated environment lacked the distractions and lighting conditions of real clinical use.

When post-market HF analysis reveals new hazards, higher-than-expected probability, or ineffective risk controls, the risk file must be re-evaluated. Hazard analysis, risk controls, and residual risk evaluations must be revised.

Why this matters: Real-world use reveals hazards no pre-market study can fully predict.

What Risk Management Actually Needs from You

Risk management needs HF engineers to understand that usability engineering and risk management are not parallel tracks. They are two perspectives on the same safety case.

Specifically, risk management needs:

- **A realistic use specification** — not just the ideal or most testable user population
- **URRA/uFMEA tightly connected to the hazard analysis**
- **Critical task identification grounded in severity from the hazard analysis**
- **Summative validation scenarios built around hazard-related use scenarios**
- **Knowledge tasks explicitly included**
- **Post-market complaint data analyzed through a use-error lens**

When HF and risk management describe the same hazards, the same tasks, the same controls, and the same evidence, the device is as safe as it can be. When they diverge, the gap between them is the risk that nobody has addressed yet.

Notes & Sources

- **On use errors, abnormal use, and reasonably foreseeable misuse** — ISO 14971:2019.
- **On the use-related risk analysis and critical task identification** — FDA, *Applying Human Factors and Usability Engineering to Medical Devices*, February 2016; FDA draft guidance, *Purpose and Content of Use-Related Risk Analyses*, July 2024.
- **On knowledge tasks and their risk management implications** — ANSI/AAMI HE75:2025, *Human Factors Engineering — Design of Medical Devices*. FDA draft guidance, *Purpose and Content of Use-Related Risk Analyses*, July 2024; ANSI/AAMI HE75:2025.

Chapter 11: Biocompatibility & Materials Science Engineering

Biocompatibility testing has a deceptively straightforward reputation in most medical device organizations. Samples are sent to a laboratory, tests are performed against a checklist of endpoints, results come back, a biological evaluation report is written, and the box is checked. If the tests pass, biocompatibility is considered complete.

This view is not entirely wrong. The testing is real, the laboratory work is rigorous, and the results matter. But this view misses the deeper truth: **biocompatibility testing is only one part of biological risk management — and by itself, it cannot conclude that all biological risks have been evaluated or controlled.**

When performed correctly, biological evaluation is a risk-management activity. It identifies biological hazards — the chemical substances in the device and their potential impact on patients. It estimates biological risk — how much of those substances patients are exposed to, under what conditions, and how that exposure compares to toxicological thresholds. It determines whether controls are adequate or whether additional controls are needed. And it feeds those conclusions directly into the device's risk management file.

When biocompatibility is treated as a standalone testing exercise rather than an integrated risk-management process, the tests may pass — but the biological risks associated with manufacturing, sterilization, supplier changes, degradation, or long-term exposure may remain unaddressed.

This chapter explains how biocompatibility engineering intersects with risk management at every stage of development — from material selection through post-market surveillance — and why each decision shapes the biological safety profile of the device.

Biological Evaluation and the Integration with Risk Management

ISO 10993-1 — the primary international standard for biological evaluation — is subtitled *"Evaluation and Testing Within a Risk Management Process."* That subtitle is not decorative. It signals that the standard is built on the same logic as ISO 14971:

- identify hazards
- analyze risks
- determine acceptability
- implement controls
- verify effectiveness

Recent and upcoming revisions of ISO 10993-1 make this alignment even more explicit, using ISO 14971 terminology such as *biological hazards*, *biologically hazardous situations*, and *biological harms*.

This means biological evaluation and ISO 14971 risk management are not two separate processes. They are the **same analytical logic applied to biological hazards**. The biological evaluation plan is part of the risk management plan. The biological evaluation report is part of the risk management file. The toxicological risk assessment is a risk estimation step.

In many organizations, these documents sit in different folders, owned in silos by different teams, reviewed through different processes. This separation creates gaps — because every decision a biocompatibility engineer makes directly affects the device's risk profile.

Why this matters: Biocompatibility is not a test. It is biological risk management.

Material Selection: Hazard Identification Starts Here

ISO 14971 activity: Hazard identification

The first and most consequential biological risk decision happens before any testing: **material selection**.

Every material that contacts the patient — directly or indirectly — is a potential source of biological hazard. Materials are chemistries. Plastics contain plasticizers, stabilizers, and dyes. Metals ionize under physiological conditions. Adhesives and coatings have their own chemical constituents. Manufacturing processes introduce residues. Sterilization creates byproducts.

The question is not whether a material is "biocompatible." The question is: What substances does this material contain, release, or generate — and what does that mean for patient exposure? For example:

- A PVC tubing historically used with DEHP may be replaced with a new plasticizer system. Same intended use, very different toxicological uncertainty.
- A polymer safe in short-term contact may not be safe for long-term implantation.
- A supplier's "biocompatible" resin may release new compounds after gamma sterilization.

Another thing to note is that a supplier's biocompatibility certificate does **not** establish the biocompatibility of the finished device. Biocompatibility applies to the device **after** molding, assembly, cleaning, and sterilization — not to raw materials.

Why this matters: Material selection defines the biological hazard profile before any test is run.

Chemical Characterization: Building the Biological Hazard Inventory

ISO 14971 activity: Hazard identification (continued) and risk estimation inputs

Once the device is in its final finished form, the next step is identifying what chemical substances it contains and what it can release in its intended use conditions.

Chemical characterization — governed by ISO 10993-18 — answers three questions:

1. What extractables can be released under aggressive laboratory conditions?
2. What leachables are released under clinical-use conditions?
3. How do extractables relate to leachables — and therefore to patient exposure?

Chemical characterization does not produce pass/fail results. It produces a **chemical inventory** — the input to toxicological risk assessment. For example:

- A device cleaned with a different detergent formulation will have a different extractables profile.
- Ethylene oxide sterilization introduces EO residuals and byproducts that must be quantified.
- A device aged to end-of-shelf-life may release different compounds than a freshly manufactured device.

Every chemical species that is identified through chemical characterization becomes a focus for toxicological analysis of the question, "How does this compound behave, given its concentration in the device matrix?" What is the lowest level above which exposure to this chemical species will lead to a significant risk?

Two key risk-based decisions

1. Thoroughness: Characterization must reflect all manufacturing steps — cleaning, bonding, molding, sterilization, aging.

2. Relevance: Extraction conditions must be representative of clinical exposure. Solvent choice, temperature, time, and surface-area ratios are scientific decisions with patient-safety implications.

Why this matters: You cannot manage biological risks that you haven't chemically identified.

Toxicological Risk Assessment: Risk Estimation for Biological Hazards

ISO 14971 activity: Risk estimation and risk evaluation

After performing the chemical analysis and having compiled an initial list of the substances, a toxicological risk assessment is conducted. Governed by ISO 10993-17, it transforms the chemical inventory into a biological risk estimate.

It is at this stage that biological hazard identification transforms into biological risk assessment, and the results obtained here become the direct source for the product risk management file.

The core tool is the **margin of safety.** Margin of safety analysis is what allows to estimate the risk involved:

- Estimate patient exposure to each substance
- Compare exposure to a toxicological threshold
- Determine whether the margin is acceptable

If the margin of safety is high, the risk is acceptable. If it is low, risk controls are required — redesign, process changes, additional cleaning, or reduced contact duration.

The toxicological risk assessment tells you which substances require action; and the risk management process determines what action is taken and whether the resulting residual risk is acceptable for the intended use.

Two areas where risk-based decisions are most critical

1. The intended patient population – Toxicological thresholds are typically based on healthy adults. But neonates, pregnant patients, immunocompromised patients, or patients with altered metabolism may have different risk profiles.

Example: A substance safe for adults at a given exposure may not be safe for neonates receiving the same device for longer durations.

2. Testing vs. analysis – ISO 10993-1 allows biological testing to be waived if chemical characterization and toxicological data sufficiently address risk. This is not a shortcut — it is a risk-based judgment. "Does the existing evidence close the biological hazard assessment with sufficient confidence for the intended use of the device, or are there gaps that only biological testing can fill?"

Why this matters: Toxicology is where biological hazard identification becomes biological risk evaluation.

Contact Categorization: Scoping the Biological Risk Assessment

ISO 14971 activity: Risk management planning — defining scope

Before or during characterization, the biocompatibility engineer must define:

- **Nature of contact:** surface-contacting, externally communicating, or implant
- **Duration of contact:** limited (<24 hours), prolonged (24 hours–30 days), or permanent (>30 days)

This is a risk-scoping decision, and it matters because getting it wrong produces a biological evaluation with incomplete biological endpoints.

The most common scoping errors involve:

- **Underestimating cumulative exposure:** A device used for 10 days per episode but used monthly for years may have *permanent* cumulative exposure.
- **Underestimating contact nature:** A "surface-contacting" device may intermittently contact mucous membranes or compromised skin, requiring additional endpoints.

The risk-based decision here is about accurately characterizing the device's actual biological hazard exposure — the full range of patient contact conditions that can reasonably be anticipated — rather than the most favorable characterization that reduces the scope of the biological evaluation program.

Why this matters: Incorrect contact categorization produces a structurally incomplete biological evaluation.

The Final Finished Form Principle: Where Most Gaps Live

Of all the concepts in this chapter, the one with the greatest practical significance for patient safety is what regulators call the **final finished form principle: Biocompatibility applies to the device exactly as it reaches the patient.** Not to raw materials. Not to subassemblies. Not to pre-sterilized components. For example:

- A polymer safe in raw form may release new compounds after injection molding due to mold-release agents.
- Gamma sterilization may cause chain scission, generating new low-molecular-weight species.
- A change in cleaning agent formulation may introduce new surface residues.

Manufacturing changes that seem unrelated to safety — such as cost reductions, supplier substitutions, process improvements — can alter the chemical profile of the final device.

The risk-based decision at every material and process change should be: "has the biological evaluation been reviewed against the changed final finished form of the device, and has the toxicological risk assessment confirmed that overall residual risk of the device remains acceptable?"

Change Control as Biological Risk Reassessment

The biological evaluation plan should define the criteria for when re-evaluation is triggered, and the biological evaluation report should be updated to reflect the conclusions of that re-evaluation. But the practical challenge is that the changes most likely to require biological re-evaluation often arrive through multiple channels. They come through:

- design changes
- supplier changes
- manufacturing process changes
- sterilization changes
- packaging changes

Each of these pathways is owned by a different function — and each can alter the final finished form.

The biocompatibility engineer's role is to ask, for every change: Does this change alter patient exposure — and what is the toxicological risk of that new exposure?

This requires visibility across functions and a change-impact process that routes relevant changes to biological risk evaluation.

Why this matters: Most biological risk gaps arise from unassessed changes.

Post-Market: Biological Risk Does Not End at Market Release

Biological evaluation is a lifecycle process. Post-market information must inform ongoing biological risk assessment.

Relevant post-market signals include:

- complaints describing adverse reactions at contact sites
- inflammatory or sensitization events
- device degradation in clinical use
- new scientific literature on material behavior

A device that passed pre-market evaluation may degrade faster in real-world conditions, releasing compounds not identified during characterization.

When post-market information indicates a change in biological risk, the biological evaluation must be updated. Hazard analysis, toxicological risk assessment, and residual risk evaluation must be revised.

This is the same lifecycle obligation that ISO 14971 establishes for all hazard categories — the risk file must stay current with real-world evidence.

Why this matters: Real-world evidence reveals biological hazards that pre-market testing cannot fully predict.

What Risk Management Actually Needs From You

Risk management needs biocompatibility and materials engineers to understand that biological evaluation **is** the risk-management process for biological hazards.

Specifically, risk management needs:

- **Material selection** treated as biological hazard identification

- **Chemical characterization** integrated with hazard analysis
- **Toxicological risk assessment** linked to the actual patient population
- **Contact categorization** that reflects real-world use
- **Final finished form evaluation** for every material and process change
- **Post-market biological surveillance** feeding back into the risk management file

The biological evaluation and the risk management file must tell the same story about the same device. When they do, the biological hazard profile is complete. When they do not, there is a system-level gap in the device's safety case.

Chapter 12: Reliability Engineering

Ask a reliability engineer what their job is, and they will tell you they make devices that work. Ask them how they know when a device works **well enough**, and most will reach for a number: mean-time-between-failures, demonstrated reliability at a given confidence level, or a target failure rate set early in development. These numbers matter — a device that fails frequently is a device that puts patients at risk.

But numbers alone cannot answer the most important question: **when the device fails, does anyone get hurt?**

A device that fails once every hundred uses may be safe if every failure triggers an alarm or forces the device into a safe state. A device that fails once every ten thousand uses may be catastrophic if that rare failure produces an incorrect output with no warning in a clinical situation where the incorrect output directly harms the patient.

Mean-time-between-failures does not distinguish between these two devices. A system-level reliability specification of 99% does not tell you whether the 1% of failures are nuisance failures or safety-critical failures. A demonstrated reliability of 99.9% at 95% confidence is a statistical achievement that says nothing about what happens to a patient when the device is in the failing 0.1%.

This is what reliability engineering lacks when it operates in a vacuum, disconnected from the risk management process.

Reliability and safety risk management are deeply intertwined. The risk management file dictates which failures matter most and how rarely they must occur for the device to be considered safe. Reliability engineering provides the tools and data to determine whether those failure-rate requirements are achievable, whether the design can meet them, and whether the device continues to meet them in the field. When this connection is missing, reliability and risk management operate in parallel — each producing documents that reference the other without truly informing it.

This chapter makes that connection explicit: what reliability engineering means for patient safety, how it interacts with the risk management file, and where the risk-based decisions live in the reliability engineer's daily work.

A Different Way to Think About Failure

Before mapping specific activities, one conceptual reframing is essential — because without it, reliability and risk management often talk past each other.

ISO 14971 is built around a two-part view of how failure becomes harm:

1. **P1:** How likely is it that a failure mode occurs and leads to a hazardous situation?
2. **P2:** How likely is it that the hazardous situation results in harm?

The probability of harm is **P1 × P2**.

Reliability engineers primarily influence **P1**. Through design decisions, component selection, stress derating, redundancy, and verification testing, they determine how likely it is that a failure mode occurs — and how likely it is that the failure, when it does occur, progresses to a hazardous situation.

This is what makes reliability engineering inherently connected to patient safety rather than merely to device performance. For instance, improving the reliability of a safety-critical function reduces P1 for the hazardous situations associated with that function's failure. This is not just performance improvement — it is **risk control at the highest level of the ISO 14971 hierarchy: inherently safe design**.

Why this matters: Reliability without hazard context can improve uptime without improving safety.

Where Reliability Requirements Come From — And Where They Should Go

Every major development program begins with reliability requirements. These often appear in design inputs and may specify:

- number of cycles without failure
- probability of successful procedure completion
- maximum allowable failure rate at a given confidence level

Where do these numbers come from?

Often from competitive benchmarking, commercial commitments, engineering tradition, or what the team believes is achievable.

But none of these sources answer the question that risk management requires:

What failure rate is acceptable for failure modes that could harm a patient?

The answer lives in two places:

1. The manufacturer's risk acceptance criteria

These criteria define which combinations of severity and probability are acceptable, acceptable only if reduced as far as possible, or unacceptable.

2. The hazard analysis

This analysis characterizes the severity of harm for each hazardous situation and patient harm.

Together, they define a **probability ceiling** for each hazardous situation — the highest probability at which the risk is still acceptable.

For example, for hazardous situations involving the most severe patient harm (such as serious injury, death, or irreversible patient damage), the acceptable probability of occurrence is very low. And for hazardous situations involving less severe patient harm, the acceptable probability rate may be higher.

These probability ceilings become **reliability targets** for the failure modes that lead to those hazardous situations.

When reliability requirements are written without reference to these ceilings, the device may meet every reliability test and still carry unacceptable patient safety risk.

Why this matters: Reliability targets that ignore risk acceptance criteria can be impressive — and still unsafe.

The Reliability Engineer's Toolkit — What Each Tool Contributes to Risk Management

Reliability engineers use a specific set of analytical tools, and each of them has a direct counterpart in the risk management process. Understanding what each tool produces in the device's risk management terms is what makes the reliability engineer a genuine contributor to the risk management file rather than a parallel practitioner. Some of those tools are discussed here, though they are not exhaustive.

1. Design Failure Modes, Effects, and Criticality Analysis (FMECA)

FMECA is a bottom-up analysis: it identifies how each component can fail, what effect that failure has, and how critical it is.

In risk management terms:

- FMECA is **hazard source identification**.
- Any failure mode that can reach a patient through a sequence of events is a **hazardous situation**.
- The "criticality" dimension bridges the failure mode to the **severity** in the hazard analysis.

Example: A capacitor failure that causes a pump motor to stall may be a nuisance in some devices — but in an infusion pump delivering vasopressors, it is a safety-critical failure mode that must be in the hazard analysis.

2. Fault Tree Analysis (FTA)

FTA is top-down. It begins with a harm or hazardous situation and maps backward to identify all combinations of failures that could produce it.

Where the DFMECA identifies what can go wrong with the components, the FTA asks how each characterized hazard can be reached from those component failures.

When component failure rates are known — from historical data, accelerated testing, or industry databases — the FTA can produce a quantitative probability estimate for the top-level event. This estimate is the most direct contribution reliability engineering can make to the probability of occurrence calculation in the risk management file.

Example: If a ventilator's "loss of ventilation" hazardous situation can be caused by three independent failures, FTA quantifies the combined probability — not just the individual failure rates.

3. Highly Accelerated Life Testing (HALT)

HALT stresses the device beyond real-world conditions to reveal design weaknesses early. This method stresses the unit under test using extreme temperature ranges, vibration, power cycles, and even combinations of all three. The purpose of this testing isn't to mimic the real world, but to stress the system beyond what could happen in reality.

In risk terms:

- HALT is **hazard identification**.
- Every failure mode discovered belongs in the FMECA.

- If it can reach a patient, it belongs in the hazard analysis.

HALT that does not feed into the risk management file produces reliability insights that never become safety insights.

Post-Market: When Field Data Changes the Risk Picture

Reliability engineering does not end at market release. In many ways, this is where its most important contribution to risk management begins.

Pre-market probability estimates are predictions — based on component data, FMECA, accelerated testing, and design analysis. Real-world use tests those predictions.

Clinical environments are more variable than test conditions. And components that performed flawlessly in controlled testing may behave differently at temperature extremes, under vibration, or in high-humidity environments.

FRACAS: The post-market reliability engine

The Failure Reporting, Analysis, and Corrective Action System (FRACAS) captures:

- field failures
- failure modes
- root causes
- corrective actions

In risk terms, FRACAS is production and post-production information required by ISO 14971.

For example: Pre-market analysis estimated a pump stall as "remote" (1 in 100,000). FRACAS shows it occurring at 1 in 5,000.

This moves the hazardous situation from acceptable to unacceptable — triggering redesign, additional controls, or revised instructions for use.

A reliability engineer who maintains FRACAS without connecting it to the risk management file is collecting data without using it for its most important purpose.

Why this matters: Field failure data is the most direct evidence of actual risk.

What Risk Management Actually Needs From You

For risk management to function effectively, reliability engineers must understand that:

- Every failure mode in the FMECA is a potential hazard source.
- Every event in the fault tree is part of a hazardous sequence.
- Every FRACAS report is evidence about the real-world probability of harm.

All of these must feed back into the risk management file. Reliability requirements written without reference to the risk file may be realistic and cost-effective — but they are disconnected from patient safety.

Reliability engineering is one of the most powerful forms of risk control available to a medical device manufacturer. Designing safety-critical functions to fail infrequently enough that hazardous situations remain within risk-acceptance criteria is an inherently safe design.

When reliability engineers understand this, their work is not just about making devices that work. It is about making devices that are safe.

Notes & Sources

- **On reliability requirements as safety design inputs** — ISO 13485:2016, Clause 7.3.3; 21 CFR 820.30.
- **On essential performance as a risk-based reliability classification** — IEC 60601-1:2005+AMD1:2012+AMD2:2020.

Chapter 13: Test Engineering (Verification & Validation)

When a verification and validation (V&V) program concludes successfully, the summary often reads: **all requirements were tested, all acceptance criteria were met, verification is complete**. What the summary does not say is whether the requirements were tested under the right conditions, whether the acceptance criteria were appropriate and risk-based, or whether the protocols were designed to demonstrate that risk controls actually work.

A medical device can pass every verification test and still have risk controls that have never been shown to function — simply because no one designed the test protocols to demonstrate their effectiveness as *risk controls*. This is one of the most common and least visible problems in medical device V&V programs. From the outside, everything appears complete: the traceability matrix is filled out, the verification reports show passing results, the risk management file references those reports, and the residual risks are assessed as acceptable. The documentation appears coherent because each artifact references the others exactly as procedures require.

But the connection to patient safety is often weaker than it appears.

The gap lives in three places:

1. **How sample sizes are chosen** — whether they reflect the consequences of failure.
2. **How test conditions are designed** — whether they reflect the scenarios in which risk controls must perform.
3. **What the team believes they are verifying** — whether they distinguish between confirming a feature exists and confirming it works when it matters.

These gaps occur when V&V is not tightly connected to the risk management file. The risk file tells the V&V engineer what matters most, what failure means in patient-safety terms, and what a test program must demonstrate to support the safety case. Without that connection, V&V still produces evidence — but not the evidence needed for patient safety.

This chapter explains the three intersections where V&V engineering and risk management meet, and the risk-based decisions that live at each one.

What V&V Engineers Actually Do — And Where Risk Management Lives in It

Verification and validation engineers design, plan, execute, and document the testing that provides objective evidence that a medical device meets its requirements. They:

- write test protocols
- define acceptance criteria
- determine sample sizes
- execute or oversee testing
- review and document results
- maintain traceability between requirements and evidence
- participate in design reviews
- respond to field data by designing additional tests

None of these tasks *automatically* require reviewing the risk management file. Requirements come from design inputs. Acceptance criteria come from specifications. Test conditions come from standards or engineering judgment. Sample sizes come from convention or past practice.

When V&V operates this way, it produces **specification-compliance evidence** — proof that the device meets its requirements. This is not sufficient. Patient safety assurance needs something more specific: **evidence that risk controls are effective** — that they actually reduce the hazardous situations they were designed to address, and to the right levels of acceptability as determined by the risk management file.

Specification compliance and risk-control effectiveness are not the same thing. A V&V program that produces the first while neglecting the second leaves the safety case resting on assumptions rather than evidence.

Why this matters: A device can meet every requirement and still fail to protect patients if the risk controls were never tested under the conditions where harm occurs.

The First Intersection: Sample Size Is a Risk-Based Decision

Every verification test requires choosing a sample size. For attribute tests (pass/fail outcomes), sample size determines the statistical confidence of the result. Passing with five samples means something very different than passing with fifty.

This is not just a statistical question. It is a risk-based decision.

Risk determines how much confidence is required:

If failure of a requirement could cause serious or irreversible harm, the test must provide strong evidence of reliability. If failure produces only minor inconvenience, the required confidence is lower.

Treating all requirements as though they need the same sample size — or choosing sample sizes by habit ("we always test 29 units") — ignores the risk management file's most fundamental output: **severity**.

Two common organizational approaches

Both are defensible:

- **Sample size tied to severity:** Higher severity → higher required reliability → larger sample size.

- **Sample size tied to overall risk level:** High-severity, high-probability hazards → most rigorous verification evidence.

Regardless of approach, the logic is the same: **Sample size must be based on the associated risk for that particular specification.**

For example: A shut-off valve that prevents overdose (severity: death) tested on five units provides weak evidence. Testing sixty units provides strong evidence. Both tests may "pass," but they do not mean the same thing.

The principle is this: the confidence and reliability level that the test needs to demonstrate — which together determine the sample size — should be proportional to the severity of the potential harm, or to the overall risk level, as defined in the risk management file (for the hazardous situation associated with the requirement being tested).

Why this matters: A small sample size for a high-severity risk control is a decision about how much uncertainty you are willing to accept about patient harm.

The Second Intersection: Test Conditions Must Reflect Hazardous Scenarios

A risk control is only as good as the conditions under which it has been shown to work.

Nominal testing — testing under standard conditions, at typical parameter values, with compliant samples — confirms that the device works as designed. It does **not** confirm that the device's safety features work under the conditions where they will be most challenged.

Risk controls are designed to prevent, detect, or mitigate specific hazardous situations. Those hazardous situations arise under specific conditions and sequence of events — as described in the hazard analysis.

Examples of hazardous-scenario conditions may include:

- elevated temperature
- electromagnetic interference
- vibration
- low battery
- power fluctuations
- maximum load
- worst-case patient physiology

A risk control that works in a quiet, temperature-controlled lab has not been shown to work in the environment where the hazardous situation actually occurs.

Worst-case testing

Worst-case testing is the V&V discipline most directly connected to risk control effectiveness. It tests the device under the harshest conditions within its intended use range — the conditions most likely to cause harm.

These conditions must come from the hazard analysis, not engineering intuition.

For example: An alarm may function perfectly at room temperature with stable power. But if the hazardous scenario occurs at high temperature and low battery, the alarm must be tested under those conditions — not just nominal ones.

Why this matters: A risk control that only works in nominal conditions has not been shown to work where patients actually get hurt.

The Third Intersection: Two Gates, Not One

ISO 14971 requires manufacturers to:

1. **Verify implementation of risk controls**, and
2. **Verify effectiveness of risk controls**.

These are not the same activity.

Gate 1: Verification of implementation

This confirms that the risk control exists in the device as designed. Examples:

- a shut-off mechanism is present
- an alarm threshold is implemented
- a software interlock is coded
- a label or warning is included

Gate 1 is necessary — but not sufficient.

Gate 2: Verification of effectiveness

This confirms that the risk control **actually reduces the hazardous situation** it was designed to address.

A risk control may be implemented correctly and still be ineffective.

For example:

- **Gate 1:** A shut-off mechanism is present and actuates correctly in the lab.
- **Gate 2:** Under real-world electromagnetic interference, the mechanism delays or fails — making it ineffective in the characterized hazardous situation.

Different controls require different evidence. For instance,

- **Design-based controls:** effectiveness shown through testing and analysis under foreseeable scenarios.
- **Protective measures (alarms, interlocks):** effectiveness shown under realistic clinical conditions.

- **Information for safety:** effectiveness shown through usability validation — not just by confirming that the label exists.

The traceability matrix that connects design inputs to design outputs to verification/validation test results to risk controls is the document that makes the two-gate structure visible:

- the control is implemented, and
- the test conditions and acceptance criteria demonstrate effectiveness.

Why this matters: A risk control that exists but has never been shown to work is a design assumption, not a safety fact.

What Risk Management Actually Needs From You

Risk management needs V&V engineers to understand that verification is not just a compliance exercise. It is the primary source of objective evidence supporting the residual risk conclusions in the risk management file.

When sample sizes are not tied to severity, when test conditions do not reflect hazardous scenarios, and when effectiveness is confused with implementation, the safety case rests on assumptions rather than evidence. And the gap between assumption and evidence is where patients are put at risk.

Risk management needs V&V engineers to review the risk management file before designing test programs — because the risk file defines what matters most, what failure means in patient-safety terms, and what a test must demonstrate to support the safety case.

A verification program built without that information may be complete on paper — but incomplete for patient safety.

Notes & Sources

- **On the requirement to verify both implementation and effectiveness of risk controls** — ISO 14971:2019.
- **On the connection between risk analysis and design inputs, including verification requirements** — ISO 13485:2016, Clauses 7.3.3 and 7.3.6.
- **On risk-based sample sizing for verification testing** — ISO 13485:2016, Clause 7.3.6.

Chapter 14: Packaging, Sterile Barrier & Sterilization Engineering

In most medical device organizations, packaging is the last thing anyone thinks about and the first thing a patient or user encounters. Packaging engineers and sterilization engineers occupy a paradoxical position in the development process: they work at the interface between design and production, at the moment when a device transitions from being engineered to being manufactured, sterilized, transported, stored, and finally opened for patient use.

These decisions are often treated as secondary — implementation details rather than safety decisions. But from the patient's perspective, they are among the most important decisions in the entire development process. A device that is brilliantly designed, correctly manufactured, and flawlessly sterilized can still harm a patient if the sterile barrier fails before it is opened, or if the package cannot be opened aseptically at the moment it is needed.

This chapter explains what packaging and sterilization engineers contribute to the risk management file — and the risk-based decisions they make every day, often without recognizing them as risk-based decisions at all.

Part One: Packaging Engineers

The Sterile Barrier As a Risk Control

For any device supplied sterile, the packaging system is not a container. It is a **risk control** — the final protective measure preventing microbial contamination from reaching the patient. The sterile barrier system (SBS), defined in ISO 11607-1 as the minimum packaging required to maintain sterility to the point of use, must simultaneously:

1. allow sterilant penetration,
2. maintain a microbial barrier through distribution and storage, and
3. enable aseptic presentation at the point of care.

Each of these functions can fail independently, and each failure represents a distinct hazardous situation that must be characterized in the risk management file.

Why this matters: If the sterile barrier fails, every upstream safety control — design, manufacturing, sterilization — fails with it.

Material Selection: Hazard Identification Starts Here

The first risk-based decision a packaging engineer makes is material selection. The material must withstand the sterilization process and the environmental stresses of the device's entire lifecycle. In making this decision, a packaging engineer either consciously or unconsciously makes a choice that can affect the patient's safety.

Different sterilization modalities impose different stresses. For example:

- **Gamma radiation** can embrittle or weaken certain polymers over time.
- **Ethylene oxide (EtO)** requires breathable materials and leaves residuals that must dissipate.
- **Steam sterilization** demands materials that tolerate high temperature and moisture.

A material may appear visually intact after sterilization but may have lost its microbial barrier properties — a failure mode invisible without proper testing.

Additionally, packaging materials must demonstrate environmental durability and remain intact across:

- temperature fluctuations during transport,
- humidity changes,
- light exposure,
- mechanical strain from handling and vibration.

For example: A pouch material that performs well at room temperature may delaminate after repeated freeze–thaw cycles during winter distribution. The seal may look intact, but the barrier is compromised — a silent failure with direct patient-safety implications.

Material selection for packaging is therefore a process of characterizing what the material will be exposed to across the device's entire journey from manufacturing to point of use and evaluating whether it will maintain its characteristics and functionality throughout that journey.

The risk analysis provides the inputs for this evaluation:

- What is the severity of harm if sterility is breached?
- What patient population is involved?
- How susceptible are they to infection?

For example: A vascular implant used in immunocompromised patients carries a higher severity than a device used in healthy outpatients — and the rigor of material qualification must reflect that.

Seal Integrity: The Risk Control That Must Not Fail at the Edges

The seal is often the weakest link in the sterile barrier system. It is where mechanical stresses concentrate during transportation, storage, and handling.

Seal integrity is evaluated through tests such as:

- bubble leak testing,
- dye penetration testing,
- seal strength testing.

These are not quality checks — they are **risk-control effectiveness tests**.

ISO 11607-1 requires packaging validation under worst-case conditions. Worst-case is not defined by what is most convenient to test, but by the conditions most likely to compromise sterility. And these **worst-case conditions must come from the hazard analysis**.

For example: A coiled device inside a peel pouch may exert localized stress on a specific seal area during vibration. A straight-configuration "worst case" would never reveal this failure mode. The true worst case is defined by the hazardous situation — not by engineering intuition.

Additionally, sample size selection for packaging validation is subject to the same risk-based principle established in the verification chapter, i.e., sample size must reflect the severity of harm associated with sterile barrier failure. A high-severity hazard requires higher reliability evidence — and therefore larger sample sizes.

Why this matters: A seal that passes nominal testing but fails under real-world stress is a risk control that has not been demonstrated to work.

Aseptic Presentation: The Risk That Appears at the Point of Use

The 2019 revision of ISO 11607-1 introduced a formal requirement for usability evaluation of aseptic presentation — demonstrating that users can open the package without contaminating the sterile contents.

This requirement formalized what clinicians had known for decades: a package that cannot be opened aseptically has failed as a risk control, regardless of how well it performed in integrity testing.

For example: An operating room nurse attempts to open a guidewire pouch during a cardiac catheterization. The peel seam tears unpredictably, causing the guidewire to "pop" out of the sterile field. The sterile barrier did not fail — the **aseptic presentation** did.

The risk-based discussion here is that the packaging design must be evaluated under realistic clinical conditions as characterized in the hazard analysis, such as gloved hands, time pressure, limited access to the package, etc.

A package that requires two people to open, or provides no clear opening start point, has failed as a risk control of contamination hazard.

Change Control: When a Packaging Change Is a Risk Management Event

Anything that is done with respect to the packaging system such as material change, new sealant machine, new package configuration, or any parameter alteration regarding the sterilization may affect the performance of the risk control of the sterile barrier. Therefore, changes in packaging systems should be considered inputs for the risk management process.

The decisions involved in the packaging change in accordance with the risk management are: Does the packaging change impact the capability of the sterile barrier as a risk control method? To answer this, one must consider whether the modification impacts the material's suitability for sterilization, the seal's integrity within the use environment, and aseptic presentation of the packaging.

In the post-market phase, packaging issues and field reports become information regarding whether the sterile barrier is functioning as intended in clinical settings. For example, complaints about damaged seals, difficulty opening pouch, etc. are post-market indications that the risk control process measures may not have been as effective in the real world as it appeared to be through validation.

Part Two: Sterilization Engineers

The Sterility Assurance Level As a Risk Acceptance Decision

The sterilization engineer's primary safety responsibility is ensuring that the device is delivered to the patient in a sterile state — with a probability of microbial survival that is acceptable according to the risk management plan.

The industry benchmark of **SAL 10^{-6}** (one-in-a-million probability of a viable microorganism) is not arbitrary. It is a **risk acceptance threshold** based on the severity of harm associated with infection.

However, the risk-based nuance here is that SAL 10^{-6} is not always sufficient — nor always necessary. For example, for implantable devices used in immunocompromised patients or in sterile body cavities, the risk assessment may justify sterility assurance beyond 10^{-6}.

And for devices with minimal patient contact, the required assurance may differ. A sterilization engineer who applies SAL 10^{-6} without referencing the hazard analysis or reviewing the characterized risks may set the wrong target.

Why this matters: SAL is not a number — it is a statement about how much infection risk the manufacturer is willing to accept.

Method Selection: Risk-Based Compatibility

Every sterilization modality affects the device, its materials, and its packaging. The risk-based question is: **can this method achieve the required SAL without creating new hazards?** Specifically, which of the device's material and functional properties are safety-critical, and what would happen to the risk profile if those properties were altered by sterilization.

For instance, Ethylene oxide (EtO) leaves toxic residuals requiring aeration and testing. And the residuals must be evaluated under ISO 10993 as part of biological risk management.

EtO compatibility links sterilization engineering directly to biocompatibility. In other words, the sterilization engineer and the biocompatibility engineer are working on the same risk question from different angles, and the risk management file is where their work must be connected.

In another instance, gamma and e-beam radiation can alter polymer properties, embrittle materials, or change surface chemistry and may weaken packaging materials or seals. The end effects must be characterized and addressed — not assumed safe.

For example: A device originally validated for gamma sterilization is later found to develop microcracks in the pouch material after dose accumulation. The sterile barrier remains visually intact but fails microbial barrier testing — a risk control failure created by the sterilization method.

Why this matters: Sterilization can eliminate microbial hazards while creating material hazards — both must be evaluated.

Validation and Re-Validation: When the Process Changes

The sterilization validation is not a one-time event. It is valid for the specific device, packaging, and manufacturing conditions that were present when the validation was conducted.

Changes to any of those elements, for example new packaging material, modified device configuration, change in manufacturing facility, supplier change for a device material, modification to the sterilization cycle parameters, etc. trigger the need to evaluate whether re-validation is required.

The risk-based decision in every change assessment is whether the change could affect the sterilization process's ability to achieve SAL 10^{-6} with the actual device and packaging system. That question cannot be answered without understanding what the original validation demonstrated. The sterilization engineer who does not comprehend the logic behind the approved parameters of the process will not be able to make sound risk-based decisions about whether changes need to be re-approved or are equivalent.

What Risk Management Actually Needs from You

Risk management needs packaging and sterilization engineers to understand that:

- The sterile barrier system is a **risk control**, not just a container for the device.
- Worst-case packaging validation must be based on the **hazard analysis**, not engineering intuition.
- Sample size must reflect the **severity of harm** associated with sterile barrier failure.
- Post-market packaging complaints are **effectiveness signals**, not quality nuisances.
- SAL 10^{-6} is a **risk acceptance decision**, not merely a universal requirement.
- Sterilization assumptions — bioburden, device configuration, packaging compatibility — are **risk management assumptions** that must be maintained throughout the device's lifecycle.

Packaging and sterilization are not downstream from safety work. They are the final steps where the device's risk controls are either preserved or lost — at the moment just before the device reaches the patient. And it is vital that all these steps are tied to the product risk management file.

Notes & Sources

- **On the packaging system as a risk control and the sterile barrier system requirements** — ISO 11607-1:2019.
- **On EtO sterilization validation and control** — ISO 11135:2014.

Chapter 15: Cybersecurity & Product Security

When a vulnerability is discovered in a connected medical device — an authentication flaw, an outdated software component, an insecure communication interface — the organizational response usually follows a predictable process. The security team evaluates the technical severity using standard security metrics. The issue is logged in the security risk register. A mitigation plan is drafted. The discussion concludes within the boundaries of the security risk management process. Meanwhile, the safety risk management file, maintained separately, remains untouched.

It is easy to understand why. Safety and security are traditionally treated as different domains, each with its own vocabulary, methods, and regulatory expectations. But for connected medical devices, this separation can be dangerous.

This chapter explains where security and safety risk management must explicitly intersect — and the risk-based decisions a product security engineer must make when a security event is also a patient safety event.

Two Processes, One Overlap

Before mapping the specific integration points, the fundamental relationship between security risk management and safety risk management needs to be stated clearly, because getting it wrong in either direction creates problems. Security risk management and safety risk management are distinct processes, but they overlap in ways that matter deeply for connected devices.

Safety risk management governs physical injury and damage to health arising from the device's design, manufacturing, and use. Security risk management governs threats to information — confidentiality, integrity, and availability — and the ways information may be exposed, modified, or made unavailable.

These domains differ in scope, analysis techniques, and time horizons. But they intersect whenever a security threat compromises a function that is safety-critical. In ISO 14971 terms, a security vulnerability becomes a **cause** of a hazardous situation when exploitation of that vulnerability impairs essential performance.

This intersection is not always obvious. For example, a buffer overflow in a logging component may have no safety relevance. The same vulnerability in a therapy-delivery module could be catastrophic.

AAMI TIR57 — the primary technical guidance for medical device security risk management — formalizes this relationship. It states that security and safety risk management run in parallel, and when a security risk has safety implications, there must be a defined pathway for communicating that risk into the safety risk management file.

For the cybersecurity engineer, the daily risk-based decision is straightforward: **does this security finding compromise a safety-critical function?** If the answer is yes, two things must happen. The safety risk management file must be revisited, and the response must be governed by both security urgency and safety risk acceptance criteria — not security urgency alone.

Integration Point One: Threat Modeling as Hazard Identification

The first place where security work must connect to safety risk management is during design, when the device architecture is being defined.

Safety risk management begins with hazard identification — a systematic search for ways the device could expose a patient to harm. Historically, this meant mechanical failures, electrical hazards, software faults, biocompatibility risks, and use errors. For connected devices, it must also include the ways an attacker could make the device behave dangerously.

Threat modeling is the security engineer's structured analysis of attack scenarios: who might attack the device, through which interfaces, using which techniques, and with what technical consequences. What threat modeling does not automatically determine is the **clinical** consequence of each scenario. That requires knowing which device functions are safety-critical — information found in the essential performance characterization and **hazard analysis**.

The integration point is simple: for each threat scenario, the security engineer must determine whether successful exploitation would compromise a safety-critical function. This requires access to the safety risk management file. When security teams and safety teams work in isolation, threat modeling becomes a purely technical exercise, and the safety implications of attack scenarios remain invisible.

Example: Why threat modeling must connect to safety

A threat model identifies a path where an attacker could modify a device's configuration logs. This has no safety impact. The same threat model identifies a path where an attacker could alter infusion pump rate calculations. This is a direct patient safety hazard. Without access to the safety-critical function list, the security engineer cannot distinguish between the two.

When a threat scenario is classified as having patient safety implications, it becomes part of the hazard analysis. It must be assigned a severity, a probability of occurrence, and a risk control. What makes security-originating hazards difficult is probability estimation. Hardware failures can be estimated using failure rate data. Security threats cannot. An intelligent adversary with knowledge and motivation can exploit a vulnerability with high certainty.

AAMI TIR57 and regulators address this by recommending that manufacturers assume **worst-case probability** for security vulnerabilities with safety implications — treat them as threats that will occur — and focus the safety evaluation on the severity of harm.

Integration Point Two: Vulnerability Findings as Risk Estimation Updates

The second integration point occurs whenever a vulnerability is discovered — during development through security testing, or post-market through disclosure or monitoring.

Once a vulnerability is identified, the security team evaluates its technical characteristics: attack surface, exploitability, and technical impact. Security frameworks can quantify these factors, but they cannot determine the **clinical** impact. That requires a safety assessment.

The key question is: **if this vulnerability were exploited, would a patient be harmed?** Answering this requires tracing the vulnerability through the device architecture — from the vulnerable component, to the function it supports, to the clinical consequence of that function failing or being manipulated.

This assessment requires the security engineer to understand which functions are safety-critical. A network communication vulnerability may be irrelevant if it affects only administrative data. The same vulnerability may be safety-critical if it affects therapy commands or alarm signaling.

If a vulnerability has patient safety implications, the response cannot follow security priorities alone. It must also follow the safety risk management file's requirements for evaluating residual risk while a patch is developed.

This creates a real tension. Security patches must be deployed urgently. But patches for medical devices must also be validated to ensure they do not introduce new safety hazards. Both urgency and safety validation are essential, and the work lies in balancing them.

Example: Patch urgency vs. safety validation

A vulnerability is discovered in a third-party library used in a ventilator's communication stack. The patch fixes the vulnerability but changes timing behavior in a way that could delay alarm transmission. The security team wants immediate deployment. The safety team requires validation. Both are right — and both constraints must be honored to ultimately ensure patient safety.

The Security Bill of Materials (SBOM) makes this assessment scalable. When a new vulnerability is disclosed in a third-party component, the SBOM allows the security engineer to immediately determine whether the component is present in the device and whether it supports safety-critical functions. Without an SBOM, this analysis must be done manually — a slow process that leaves devices exposed during the window between disclosure and patch availability.

Integration Point Three: Post-Market Monitoring as Production and Post-Production Information

ISO 14971 requires manufacturers to systematically collect and review production and post-production information that could affect the risk management file. For connected devices, the most important source of this information is post-market security monitoring.

This includes:

- newly disclosed vulnerabilities in software components,
- intelligence from security researchers and coordinated disclosure programs,
- security incidents in the broader healthcare ecosystem.

Every disclosed vulnerability affecting a component listed in the SBOM is potential production and post-production information. ISO 14971 requires asking whether this new information affects the probability or severity of any hazardous situation or if it identifies uncharacterized safety risks. If it does, the risk management file must be updated and residual risk re-evaluated.

The **risk-based** decision here is **triage**: of all disclosed vulnerabilities, which ones have safety implications that require immediate action? This triage requires joint analysis: whether the component is present, whether the affected function is safety-critical, and whether exploitation would create or worsen a hazardous situation.

Post-market security surveillance also keeps the threat model current. The threat environment evolves as new attack methods emerge, as healthcare networks change, and as researchers examine devices long after release. A threat model that was complete at launch may be inadequate years later. It must be reviewed periodically, and the safety risk management file must be re-evaluated when new threats create new avenues for patient harm.

What Risk Management Actually Needs from You

Risk management needs product security engineers to understand that every threat scenario, every vulnerability finding, and every post-market security signal may have patient safety implications — and that determining whether it does requires understanding the safety risk management file. It needs:

- Threat modeling to classify each attack scenario against the device's safety-critical functions and essential performance.
- Vulnerability assessments to be triaged not only through security frameworks but also through safety risk criteria (a vulnerability's CVSS score indicates technical severity; it does not indicate clinical consequence).
- Post-market security monitoring to be formally connected to ISO 14971's production and post-production information review.

Security and safety risk management can be separate processes. But for connected devices, they cannot afford to be strangers.

Notes & Sources

- **On the distinct but overlapping relationship between security risk management and safety risk management** — AAMI TIR57:2016/(R)2023; FDA, *Cybersecurity in Medical Devices*, 2023/2025.
- **On the communication pathway between security and safety risk processes** — ANSI/AAMI SW96:2023.
- **On post-market security monitoring as production and post-production information** — AAMI TIR97:2019/(R)2023.
- **On the Software Bill of Materials as a post-market risk management tool** — FDA, *Cybersecurity in Medical Devices*, 2023/2025.

Part III — Quality, Supply Chain & Manufacturing

Chapter 16: Quality Assurance & Quality Systems

Most medical device manufacturers have ISO 14971-compliant risk management files, documented risk acceptance criteria, and risk management reports signed before product release. They also maintain mature quality management systems with procedures for nonconformance disposition, CAPA, change control, supplier qualification, internal audits, and management review.

What many organizations lack is integration between these two systems. Risk acceptance criteria defined in the risk management plan often do not appear in the QMS procedures that govern daily decisions. A CAPA triage process may use a ranking system that has no relationship to the product's safety risk. A nonconformance disposition process may rely on engineering judgment without referencing the risk documented in the hazard analysis.

This is a governance problem. A risk-based quality system does not mean having both a risk management process and a QMS. It means that the risk acceptance criteria established by top management under ISO 14971 govern the decisions made every day throughout the QMS. The rigor of each QMS process must be proportionate and commensurate with the product safety risk it touches.

This chapter is for quality leaders and quality systems engineers who own this connection — and who are responsible for embedding it into procedures, decisions, and organizational culture.

What a Risk Policy Actually Is — and Why It Matters

ISO 14971 requires top management to establish a risk policy: a documented statement of the organization's approach to risk and the criteria for risk acceptability. Most organizations have such a policy. It defines severity and probability categories, the risk matrix, and the thresholds for acceptability, reduction, or benefit-risk justification.

What happens to the risk policy after it is written is the central question of this chapter.

In a risk-based quality system, the risk policy is the **constitutional document** for patient safety decisions. It governs not only what goes into the risk management file but also every risk-relevant decision made throughout the device lifecycle. A nonconformance disposition is a risk acceptance decision. A change control assessment is a safety risk evaluation. Supplier audit frequency is a product risk classification decision. Each of these activities makes a judgment about whether a deviation, change, or gap reaches a threshold requiring action to ensure the device remains safe.

When the link to product risk is missing, each QMS process develops its own prioritization criteria, escalation rules, and definitions of urgency. The organization ends up running multiple parallel risk acceptance strategies with no assurance that they align with each other — or with patient safety.

Quality leaders seeking to implement a risk-based QMS can begin with a simple audit: **Do the criteria from the risk management file clearly dictate how we triage CAPAs, disposition nonconformances, assess changes, qualify suppliers, plan audits, and prepare management review?**

The FDA's QMSR Makes It Explicit

The FDA's Quality Management System Regulation (QMSR), effective February 2, 2026, incorporates ISO 13485:2016 by reference and makes the expectation of risk-based QMS processes explicit. The previous Quality System Regulation mentioned risk only in design validation. ISO 13485 integrates risk throughout the QMS — in planning, product realization, purchasing controls, production and service provision, monitoring and measurement, and feedback processes.

The QMSR's preamble is direct: risk management is expected throughout the quality system, not confined to design. This is not new in spirit — FDA's 1996 QSR intended risk-based thinking even without using the terminology — but it is now a documented requirement.

Quality systems engineers updating procedures should ask: **What is the risk-based decision in this process, and where is the connection to the product's risk management file?**

Nonconformance Disposition: The Daily Risk Decision

One of the most frequent risk-based decisions in a medical device company occurs at the Material Review Board, where quality engineers disposition nonconforming product. Should it be used as-is, reworked, or scrapped? These decisions are made constantly, often under time pressure, and often without reference to the risk management file.

This is significant because nonconformance is not only a quality issue — it is a safety question. The disposition depends on what the nonconforming attribute affects. Some specifications are aesthetic and have no safety relevance.

For example, there may be some specifications which are merely aesthetic in nature such as the appearance of the housing or color uniformity of the indicator. Failure of the product to conform to the specified requirement will not affect patient safety. But others exist solely to fulfill a risk control: for example, minimum bond strength to prevent tip detachment, burst pressure thresholds, or dimensional tolerances that ensure safe function. Deviating from these specifications is a **risk acceptance decision**, not a quality preference.

Quality leaders must build this linkage proactively. Every nonconformance requiring disposition for a finished device or critical component should include a defined step: identify whether the nonconforming characteristic corresponds to critical failure mode or a risk control in the risk management file, and evaluate the disposition against the risk acceptance criteria.

The rigor of nonconformance disposition must be **commensurate with the product safety risk** of the affected characteristic.

CAPA: When the Problem Is a Patient Safety Signal

CAPA addresses systemic issues — patterns and root causes that require correction or prevention. The question for this chapter is not how to conduct a root cause analysis, but **how the risk management file determines which problems warrant a CAPA and how urgently.**

The risk level characterization in the risk management file should govern CAPA prioritization. A complaint about an incorrect clinical reading is categorically different from a complaint about a cosmetic scratch. Both may enter the same QMS process, but the risk management file distinguishes one as safety-critical and the other as cosmetic. That distinction should determine whether a CAPA is opened, its priority, and its required resolution timeframe.

If an organization uses the same criteria for all CAPAs regardless of patient safety impact, it has disconnected its corrective action process from its risk management process. The result is predictable: resources are spent solving low-priority issues with the same rigor as high-priority ones, while safety-critical problems may go unaddressed.

A risk-oriented CAPA process begins with two questions: **What is the potential severity of harm if the root cause persists? Does the trend indicate a shift in probability that would change the residual risk conclusion?**

When a CAPA identifies a systemic root cause that undermines a risk control — for example, a process repeatedly producing bond strength out of specification, an inspection step failing to detect a critical property, or a software build process omitting a safety requirement — the CAPA effectiveness verification is identical to risk control effectiveness verification under ISO 14971.

Closing a CAPA for a safety-critical issue requires verifying the effectiveness of the risk control thoroughly (proportional to the level of risk) — not merely fixing the process. This topic is discussed in further detail in Chapter 18.

Change Control: Every Change Is a Risk Management Event

Design changes, manufacturing changes, supplier changes, labeling changes — change control is the mechanism that ensures modifications do not introduce new risks or compromise existing risk controls. This topic appears throughout the book because every function touches it.

Yet change control assessments often focus on regulatory impact (submission, supplement, notification) and procedural impact (re-validation, training, document updates), while the patient safety question — **does this change affect product risk?** — is often overlooked.

The risk-based decision in change control mirrors nonconformance disposition, but prospectively: Does the proposed change affect a characteristic identified as a risk control? Does it introduce new risks or alter the device's risk profile?

A change to a sealing parameter may affect sterile barrier integrity. A software update may affect alarm timing. A material substitution may affect biocompatibility. These assessments cannot be made without referencing the risk management file.

Quality systems engineers who own change control procedures should ensure that every change assessment form includes a defined pathway to the risk management file — not a generic question about risk impact, but a specific requirement to identify what exactly has (or has not) been impacted with regards to patient safety decisions.

And the following design controls rigor must be proportionate to the safety impact of the affected characteristic.

Document Control: Not All Documents Carry the Same Safety Weight

Document control is often treated as an administrative function — version management, approvals, and archival. In a risk-based QMS, it is a safety function.

Work instructions, test methods, and specifications that implement or verify risk controls carry a different safety weight than documents governing non-critical activities. Changes to these documents require more rigorous and frequent review, cross-functional approval, and sometimes safety validation. The risk management file should inform which documents fall into this category.

Document control rigor must be commensurate with the product safety risk associated with the document's content.

Training and Competence: Rigor Where It Matters Most

Training is another QMS process that must be proportional to product safety risk. Tasks that implement or verify safety-critical functions — for example, sealing processes for sterile barriers, inspection of safety-critical components, software testing for essential performance — require more rigorous training, qualification, and periodic re-assessment than those tasks that do not directly affect patient safety.

And if this book makes one point clear, it is that everyone in a medical device organization influences patient safety in some way — and that certain tasks demand a higher level of training and rigor than others for all of us.

The risk management file should identify which work instructions and roles require elevated training rigor.

Supplier Qualification: Criticality Comes from the Risk Management File

Manufacturers are responsible for patient safety regardless of how many components are sourced externally. Supplier quality management extends this responsibility into the supply chain and the risk-based question in supplier management is: how much oversight does each supplier require, and what determines that level?

Most organizations have some form of supplier risk classification — a tiering system that distinguishes critical suppliers from approved suppliers from general suppliers. The classification criteria vary, but they typically include some combination of whether:

- the component is safety-critical or performance-critical,
- the supplier is sole-sourced, and
- the component requires incoming inspection or can be dock-to-stock.

What the classification criteria less commonly include is explicit reference to the risk management file for identifying the safety-critical components.

This is the connection that makes supplier qualification genuinely risk-based. A component that is the **physical implementation of a risk control**, for example a valve that prevents over-pressurization, a sensor that detects a life-threatening condition, a polymer formulation that provides the biocompatible patient-contacting surface, should receive the highest level of supplier qualification rigor and the most intensive ongoing monitoring, because its quality performance directly determines whether the risk control is effective in the field. Supplier oversight must be proportionate to the safety impact of the component.

Translating this into supplier management practice means the risk management file should be an input to supplier classification.

It also means that supplier changes carry the same risk management obligations as design changes. A substitution for a critical component requires evaluating whether the risk control's effectiveness is maintained. This topic is further discussed in Chapter 20.

Production and Process Controls: Rigor Proportionate to Safety Impact

Production and process controls — including process validation — are covered in depth in Chapter 17. The principle here is simple: processes that produce or verify safety-critical characteristics must be validated, monitored, and audited with rigor proportionate to the severity of harm they are intended to prevent.

Internal Audit: Risk-Based Planning and Risk-Informed Findings

Internal audit verifies that processes operate as intended. Most audit programs plan coverage based on regulatory requirements and process maturity. Both are valid, but neither ensures that audit resources focus on processes with the greatest patient safety impact.

The missing input is the risk management file.

Processes that implement or monitor risk controls for high-severity hazardous situations carry a different safety weight than those that do not. Audit planning should ask: **Which processes, if operating outside their defined parameters, would cause the device to exceed the acceptance criteria in the risk management file?**

The answer to this question informs the depth, frequency, and focus of audit activity within that coverage to ensure that the quality system processes are consistently delivering safe products to patients and users.

The risk management file is one of the references that makes audit planning genuinely risk-based and audit findings genuinely patient-safety-informed. Building the habit of consulting it — before planning each audit cycle and before classifying each significant finding — is the organizational practice that connects the audit program to the patient safety system it is supposed to be verifying.

Bottom line: audit depth, frequency, and focus must be commensurate with the product safety risk associated with each process.

Management Review: Risk Metrics, Not Quality Metrics

Management review is where leadership evaluates the QMS and makes decisions about resources and priorities. Most organizations present quality metrics — complaint volumes, CAPA cycle times, audit findings, supplier performance.

In a risk-based QMS, management review must present **patient safety signals**, interpreted through the risk management file.

Quality metrics are volume-neutral with respect to safety. A high volume of cosmetic complaints and a low volume of alarm failures appear similar unless mapped to severity. Complaint trends should be analyzed by device function and mapped to the hazard analysis. Nonconformance patterns should be evaluated for whether they correspond to risk controls. CAPA performance should distinguish safety-critical CAPAs from general ones. Audit findings in safety-critical processes should be highlighted separately.

This mapping gives leadership the information needed to make decisions grounded in patient safety, not just quality system performance.

What Risk Management Actually Needs from You

Risk management needs quality leaders to understand that a true risk-based QMS exists only when the organization's risk policy and risk acceptance criteria visibly govern daily decisions in nonconformance disposition, CAPA triage, change control, supplier management, document control, training, internal audit, production controls, and management review.

Every QMS process that makes a risk-relevant decision must have a defined pathway to the risk management file. The quality management system is the infrastructure through which the patient safety commitments made in the risk management file are either honored or abandoned.

A risk policy that governs the risk management file but not the QMS is a policy in name only. A quality leader who builds this governance throughout the organization is fulfilling the purpose of the risk management framework itself.

Notes & Sources

- **On the integration of risk management throughout the quality management system** — ISO 13485:2016; 21 CFR Part 820 (QMSR), effective February 2, 2026.
- **On nonconformance, CAPA, change control, and audit as risk management activities** — ISO 14971:2019; ISO 13485:2016, Clauses 8.2.2, 8.3, 8.5.

Chapter 17: Manufacturing Engineering & Process Development

Ask a manufacturing engineer what a process FMEA is for, and most will give a similar answer: it identifies where the process could fail, prioritizes those failures using the risk priority number, and drives actions to reduce the highest-priority risks. This answer is correct. It is also incomplete in a way that matters enormously for patient safety.

A process FMEA, as typically conducted, is a manufacturing quality tool. It asks what can go wrong in the process, how severe the consequence would be for the product, how often it might occur, and how detectable it would be. The outputs are process-level priorities — which failure modes need better controls, tighter parameters, or more inspection. This is valuable work. But it operates almost entirely within the manufacturing domain, with minimal consideration of patient safety.

What the pFMEA rarely asks is: Which of these process failure modes correspond to hazardous situations already characterized in the product's safety risk management file? Which failures would cause or contribute to harm reaching a patient — not just nonconforming product reaching the next assembly step? When that question is asked, and when the manufacturing engineer reads the risk management file to answer it, the pFMEA changes character. It stops being a manufacturing quality tool and becomes the manufacturing engineer's contribution to patient safety.

This chapter is about that connection — the specific places where the manufacturing engineer's daily work intersects with the product safety risk management file, and what risk-based decisions look like when those intersections are understood.

Design Transfer: Inheriting the Risk Management File

Design transfer is the moment when the design team's work becomes the manufacturing team's responsibility. The design history file moves from R&D to operations — work instructions are written, equipment is qualified, the process is validated, and production begins.

What most organizations transfer during design transfer is the specification. Dimensions, tolerances, material requirements, performance criteria, inspection methods. The assumption embedded in this transfer is that if the process consistently meets the specification, the product is safe.

But the manufacturing engineer's first responsibility at design transfer is to familiarize with the **risk management file**, not the specification alone. The risk management file answers a question the specification cannot: Which characteristics are **risk controls**, and what happens to a patient if this characteristic falls outside its **acceptable range** in a delivered device? A cosmetic tolerance and a mechanical barrier preventing device fracture may look identical on a drawing. Only the risk management file distinguishes them.

Once the manufacturing engineer knows which process steps create characteristics that serve as risk controls, the design of those steps — equipment, parameters, and controls — is driven by more than producibility. The question becomes: Can this process produce this risk control reliably, even under worst-case production conditions — human variability, material variability, equipment variability — so that the hazard is truly controlled?

Process validation as verification of risk control effectiveness: Process validation is how manufacturing engineers answer that question with objective evidence. Widely used process validation guidance originating from GHTF (now IMDRF) states that *"process validation may be considered a type of verification of the effectiveness of a risk control."* When a manufacturing engineer validates a sealing process that ensures sterile barrier integrity, they are not merely proving that the process can achieve the desired outcome. They are demonstrating that the microbial contamination risk control has been effectively implemented in production.

Process validation is no longer about meeting a regulatory requirement. It is about providing the evidence needed for product risk management.

Why this matters: A manufacturing process that produces a characteristic associated with a high-severity hazardous situation must be validated with rigor commensurate with the severity of harm. The risk management file's severity characterization makes this allocation rational rather than conventional.

Manufacturing As an Additional Layer of Risk Reduction.

Design transfer is also an opportunity that many manufacturing engineers overlook: the opportunity to ask whether the production process can add risk reduction beyond what the design specification requires.

The ISO 14971 risk control hierarchy — inherent safety, protective measures, information for safety — does not end at the design team's door. Some of the most important risk controls in a device's safety case are implemented entirely in manufacturing. For example, sterilization processes eliminate biological contamination; inspection steps remove nonconforming units before they reach patients. These are manufacturing-introduced protective measures, and they can be designed intentionally rather than by convention.

The pFMEA's Real Job

A well-executed pFMEA maps the manufacturing process's failure modes and their consequences. This is valuable, but it becomes genuinely meaningful for patient safety only when those failure modes are connected to the hazardous situations in the risk management file.

Most pFMEAs are conducted without this connection. The team identifies failures in manufacturing terms: a welding failure produces a weak joint; a sterilization failure leaves residual contamination; a measurement error allows an out-of-spec component to pass. And the severity in the FMEA is assessed based on product quality impact, not patient safety.

The missing question is: If this failure mode results in a delivered device, what is the patient safety consequence? And does that consequence correspond to a hazardous situation already characterized in the risk management file?

When the pFMEA is conducted with the hazard analysis in hand, each failure mode is assessed differently. A sterilization failure is no longer just a quality issue if inadequate surface preparation corresponds to a biological hazard with high-severity consequences. It becomes a patient safety issue, and the process controls designed to prevent it carry a different weight.

This connection transforms the pFMEA from a manufacturing document into a patient safety document.

Manufacturing data validates — or invalidates — design assumptions: The pFMEA also generates information that the risk management file's probability estimates may have assumed without verifying. Design risk estimates often assume a certain process capability. Those assumptions are only as valid as the manufacturing process's actual performance.

When the pFMEA identifies a failure mode with a defect rate higher than the assumption embedded in the risk management file, the residual risk conclusion may no longer be valid. The probability of the hazardous situation occurring may be higher than estimated.

Why this matters: Manufacturing is the primary generator of real-world probability data. When process data, inspection results, or CAPA investigations show that a failure mode is occurring more frequently than anticipated, the appropriate response is not only to strengthen process controls — but also to revisit the risk management file's probability estimates and residual risk conclusions.

In-Process Inspection: Risk Control Monitoring, Not Just Quality Gating

Every manufacturing line has inspection steps — checkpoints that prevent nonconforming product from advancing. For most characteristics, this is a quality control activity. A cosmetic inspection step that catches scratches is a quality gate, and sampling plans can be chosen based on cost and efficiency.

But for **safety-critical characteristics**, inspection is not just quality control. It is **risk control monitoring**. Its purpose is to protect patients from receiving a compromised device.

This distinction changes how inspection must be designed. The governing question becomes: What level of nonconforming product escape is acceptable for this characteristic, given that each escaped unit potentially delivers a compromised device to a patient?

For high-severity hazardous situations, the acceptable escape rate is a **risk acceptance decision** governed by the risk management file. In some cases, this means inspecting every unit instead of a sample — because sampling plans that are appropriate for non-critical characteristics may allow escape rates that are unacceptable for safety-critical elements.

Process Change and Production Data: The Manufacturing Engineer's Ongoing Contribution

Manufacturing processes evolve. Equipment wears. Parameters are adjusted. Suppliers change materials. Work instructions are revised. Each change has the potential to alter whether the process continues to reliably produce risk controls.

ISO 14971 Clause 10 requires systematic review of production and post-production information. Manufacturing engineers generate most of this information: yield trends, nonconformance rates, capability data, inspection results. These signals tell the risk management team whether the process continues to reliably implement the risk control measures that the design team specified.

When yield declines on a safety-critical step, or when nonconformance rates trend upward, or when capability data drifts toward a limit — these are not just quality signals. They may indicate an increased probability of a hazardous situation, meaning the risk management file no longer reflects reality.

A manufacturing engineer who recognizes this is not merely collecting data. They are providing the real-time safety intelligence that the risk management file depends on.

What Risk Management Actually Needs from You

Risk management needs manufacturing engineers to:

- **Understand the risk management file at design transfer** The specification tells you what to produce. The risk management file tells you why it matters — which characteristics are safety-critical and what harm follows if they fail.
- **Design and validate processes with rigor proportionate to severity** High-severity risk controls require validation and monitoring at a level commensurate with their safety impact.
- **Conduct pFMEAs with the hazard analysis in hand** A failure mode's patient safety consequence determines its true priority.
- **Treat inspection of safety-critical characteristics as risk control monitoring** Sampling plans appropriate for cosmetic features are not appropriate for safety-critical features.
- **Evaluate process changes through the lens of patient safety** Every change must be assessed for its impact to product risk and ultimately patient safety.
- **Feed production data into the risk management file** Yield trends, capability studies, and nonconformance patterns are real-world probability inputs that keep the risk file accurate.

Manufacturing is the last place where a device's risk controls can be strengthened before it reaches the patient — and the place where those controls can be silently compromised.

Closing that gap is the manufacturing engineer's most important contribution to patient safety, and it begins with understanding the risk management file.

Notes & Sources

- **On process validation as verification of risk control effectiveness** — GHTF/SG3/N99-10:2004, *Quality Management Systems — Process Validation Guidance* (Edition 2).
- **On design transfer and the connection between design outputs and manufacturing process controls** — ISO 13485:2016, Clause 7.3.8.

Chapter 18: CAPA (Corrective Action, Preventive Action)

In most medical device companies, the CAPA system is the institutional memory of the quality management system — the mechanism used to identify the source of issues, determine root cause, and implement changes systematically so that problems do not recur. Quality engineers know the steps well: initiation, containment, investigation, correction, corrective action, verification of effectiveness, closure.

But whenever a CAPA is initiated — for a nonconformity, a complaint trend, or a process deviation — one question must guide every subsequent decision: Will this problem, as it has occurred, result in a hazardous situation? The urgency, scope, and depth of the CAPA must be proportionate and commensurate with the **patient safety impact** of that failure mode.

If the answer is yes — if the defect, failure, or deviation corresponds to a failure mode that the risk management file identifies as contributing to patient harm — then the CAPA is automatically a patient safety response, not merely a quality system activity.

This chapter is short because the core argument is simple: every decision within a CAPA — containment, safety impact assessment, corrective action scope, effectiveness verification — must be risk-based and governed by the risk management file's characterization of patient safety impact, not by quality system convention alone.

The Safety Question Every CAPA Must Answer

Every CAPA must begin with a defined role — whether the CAPA owner, the quality specialist, or the risk management engineer — who opens the hazard analysis and asks: Does the failure mode described in this CAPA correspond to a hazardous situation in the risk management file? If so, what is the severity of patient harm if that hazardous situation occurs? If not, should it be newly characterized?

The answer to this question determines everything that follows. If the CAPA problem corresponds to a hazardous situation characterized at high severity — if the failure mode is a cause of patient harm — then the investigation is a patient safety investigation. Its urgency, scope, corrective action requirements, and effectiveness thresholds must be proportionate to that severity of harm.

Why this matters: A CAPA that treats a safety-critical failure mode as a routine quality issue will under-contain, under-investigate, and under-correct — leaving future patients exposed to preventable harm.

ISO 14971 Clause 10 makes this obligation explicit. It requires that production and post-production information — for which CAPA is a primary vehicle — be reviewed to determine whether:

- previously unrecognized hazards have been introduced,
- the estimated risk of a hazardous situation is no longer acceptable,
- the overall residual risk is no longer acceptable, or
- the original risk assessment has been invalidated.

In practice, many organizations do not perform this review consistently. The organizations that get it right have defined checkpoints — early in the CAPA and throughout its lifecycle — where the risk management file is consulted and the patient safety implications are explicitly assessed.

Containment As a Risk Acceptance Decision

Containment is the immediate action taken to prevent a problem from spreading before the root cause is understood. It may involve holding inventory, quarantining in-process product, suspending a process step, or communicating with field teams. These decisions are made under time pressure and with incomplete information.

Because containment is made under uncertainty, it is inherently a **risk acceptance decision**.

A manufacturer who contains broadly — quarantining all potentially affected lots or suspending production — accepts the cost and disruption of over-containment to ensure that no patient receives a potentially unsafe device. A manufacturer who contains narrowly — holding only the directly implicated lot — accepts the risk that additional affected product may be in the field or production stream.

The risk management file's severity characterization is the most important input to this decision.

- For high-severity hazards — serious, irreversible, or life-threatening — broad containment, early field communication, and suspension of distribution may be appropriate.
- For moderate severity hazards, containment may be narrower but must be reassessed as information develops.
- For minor or negligible hazards, narrower containment may be acceptable while the investigation proceeds at proportionate urgency.

Most CAPA containment decisions are made by asking: **What product is definitely affected?** The better question is: **What product might be affected, and what is the patient safety consequence if it is — and we did not contain it?**

Field Containment: Containment decisions extend beyond product in-house. A failure mode with high-severity consequences may require early communication to healthcare providers or patients even before the investigation is complete — because the patient safety risk of continued exposure outweighs the regulatory or reputational risk of communicating prematurely.

The risk management file's characterization of the hazardous situation — the patient population at risk, the severity and reversibility of harm, and the conditions under which harm occurs — is the primary input to field containment decisions. Field action decisions are discussed in further detail in Chapter 28.

Corrective Action and Effectiveness as Patient Safety Obligations

A corrective action that updates a work instruction, retrains personnel, or adds a quality check may address a quality system problem. But for a failure mode with high-severity patient consequences, these actions are rarely sufficient on their own.

For safety-relevant problems, the adequacy of corrective action is established by demonstrating that the **specific failure mode that exposes the patient to harm has been eliminated at its root**. This may require:

- a design change,
- a manufacturing process change,
- a supplier qualification change, or
- a field action for product already distributed.

Procedure updates and retraining may be part of the response, but they are not the only response.

Correction vs. Corrective Action: This distinction is meaningful for patient safety:

A **correction** addresses the immediate instance — quarantining a batch, scrapping units, resolving the deviation.

A **corrective action** addresses the systemic cause — why it happened in a way that could happen again, and what has to be changed so that it cannot.

For high-severity failure modes, a correction alone — even a well-executed one — leaves future patients exposed until the systemic cause is eliminated.

Effectiveness Verification: Effectiveness verification is the final obligation of the CAPA process. For a safety-relevant CAPA, the effectiveness check must measure **whether the failure mode has actually been reduced or mitigated**, not merely whether the corrective action plan was followed.

An effectiveness check that confirms a procedure was implemented but does not measure whether the failure mode has been mitigated has only verified compliance — not safety.

What Risk Management Actually Needs from You

Risk management needs CAPA engineers and quality professionals to:

- **Recognize that every CAPA is a potential patient safety investigation** This determination requires referencing the risk management file, not relying on intuition or quality conventions.
- **Make containment decisions governed by severity** The acceptable risk of under-containment must be proportionate to the severity of harm associated with the hazardous situation.
- **Conduct safety impact assessments using the risk management file** Internal assessments must align with the risk file's characterization of the failure mode; misalignment leads to corrective actions that are not commensurate with true risk.
- **Ensure corrective actions eliminate the systemic cause of safety-relevant failures**.
- **Verify effectiveness by measuring risk reduction, not procedural compliance** The question is not "Was the action implemented?" but "Did the failure mode stop occurring?"

The CAPA system is the quality organization's most powerful mechanism for catching failures before they reach the field — or for responding when they already have. That power depends entirely on asking the right question from the start: **What does this problem mean for the patients who depend on this device?**

Chapter 19: Metrology & Calibration

In most medical device manufacturing organizations, calibration is understood as a compliance program. Equipment is calibrated on schedule, records are maintained, and out-of-tolerance findings are documented and corrected. For example, a calibration label on a gauge or probe signals to auditors that the measurement system has been verified against a traceable standard. It signals to the quality system that the equipment is approved for use.

What the calibration label does **not** tell the organization is what the instrument's measurements are actually confirming — or whether the accuracy and frequency of calibration are adequate for the **patient safety implications** of that measurement.

A torque wrench used to assemble a cosmetic housing cover and a torque wrench used to assemble a connector that must remain secure during a cardiac monitoring procedure are both calibrated instruments. They are on the same calibration schedule, maintained under the same program, and labeled with the same status. Yet their roles are fundamentally different. One ensures cosmetic conformance. The other verifies a **risk control** essential to patient monitoring.

This chapter highlights that difference. Metrologists and calibration engineers must ensure that measurements remain true throughout the device's production and service life — especially when those measurements confirm safety-critical characteristics.

Not All Measurements Are Equal

The first link between metrology and patient safety is simple: **not all measurements carry the same safety weight**. Some measurements confirm cosmetic or performance attributes. Others confirm risk controls that prevent hazardous situations.

A risk-based calibration program begins with classification: Which instruments measure risk controls, and what level of patient harm would occur if those instruments were incorrect? This is not a complex analysis. It is a mapping exercise — but it is the foundation for a calibration program that is **commensurate with product safety risk**.

Measurement Uncertainty as a patient safety consideration: Every measurement has uncertainty. In many organizations, uncertainty is treated as a technical detail of calibration rather than a patient safety issue. But when an instrument measures a safety-critical characteristic, uncertainty becomes a direct safety question: Is the measurement system precise enough to confirm that the safety-critical characteristic is truly within its acceptable range?

If the measurement uncertainty is large relative to the tolerance band of a safety-critical characteristic, the instrument cannot reliably confirm that the risk control measure works — even if it is "in calibration" on paper.

Why this matters: A measurement system that cannot distinguish between conforming and nonconforming values for a safety-critical characteristic is not a risk control. It is a blind spot.

When an Instrument Is Found Out of Tolerance: The Patient Safety Obligation

When a calibrated instrument is found outside its tolerance limits at a scheduled calibration check — an out-of-tolerance (OOT) finding — the compliance response is straightforward: recalibrate the instrument, document the finding, and initiate corrective action. This is necessary.

But the **patient safety response** requires an additional step that many organizations treat as an afterthought: a retrospective review of all measurements made by the out-of-tolerance instrument since its last known good calibration.

ISO 13485:2016, Clause 7.6, makes this obligation explicit: when monitoring and measurement equipment is found not to conform to requirements, the organization must assess and record the validity of previous measuring results. This is not optional.

Yet in practice, retrospective reviews often become documentation exercises: a record is created, the interval of potential impact is noted, and the review concludes that no affected products can be identified or that the drift was unlikely to cause nonconformance.

But the real question is not whether documentation exists. The real question is: What did this instrument measure since its last good calibration — and did any of those measurements confirm safety-critical characteristics?

If the out-of-tolerance instrument measured safety-critical features — torque on safety-critical fasteners, sterilization cycle temperature, or any characteristic tied to a risk control — an additional assessment is required:

- What is the severity of the hazardous situation managed by this risk control?
- Given the magnitude and direction of the calibration drift, is it plausible that the instrument falsely confirmed conformance for products that were actually nonconforming?

This risk characterization determines what happens next. For high-severity hazardous situations, the response must be **proportionate as such**: lot quarantine, patient safety impact assessment, potential field action. For low-severity hazards, a documented assessment and enhanced monitoring may be sufficient.

Why this matters: An out-of-tolerance instrument that measures a safety-critical characteristic is not a paperwork issue. It is a potential patient safety event.

Organizations that navigate this well are those that have already mapped which instruments measure safety-critical characteristics — so that when an OOT finding occurs, the safety question can be answered immediately.

Beyond the Manufacturing Floor: Service, Installation, and Field Tools

Calibration obligations do not end at the manufacturing floor. Devices installed, serviced, or repaired in the field rely on measurements made with tools belonging to the service organization's calibration program. When those tools measure safety-critical characteristics, they carry the same patient safety obligations as manufacturing instruments.

This is a common organizational gap. Manufacturing metrology and field service calibration are often managed by different teams, with different rigor, documentation standards, and oversight intensity. The manufacturing program may be risk-classified and robust. The service program may be calendar-based and undifferentiated.

But the **risk** does not change simply because the measurement occurs outside the manufacturing site. ISO 14971's scope extends through the device lifecycle, including installation and servicing. If a service procedure verifies or restores a safety-critical characteristic, the tools used must be calibrated with **rigor** commensurate with the risk of the associated hazardous situation.

Service engineers and field calibration owners who reference the risk management file play a critical role in extending patient safety thinking across the entire device lifecycle.

Why this matters: A device that is safe at release but misadjusted in the field by an uncalibrated tool is no longer within the risk profile documented in the risk management file.

What Risk Management Actually Needs from You

Risk management needs metrology and calibration engineers to:

- **Recognize calibration as a patient safety function** Every instrument measuring a safety-critical characteristic confirms the presence of a risk control measure.
- **Classify instruments based on the risk controls they verify** Calibration frequency, tolerance limits, and OOT response must be **commensurate with the risk.**
- **Treat measurement uncertainty as a safety question** A measurement system must be precise enough to confirm that a risk control is truly in place.
- **Conduct OOT reviews as patient safety assessments** The question is not "Was the review documented?" but "Did this drift compromise a safety-critical characteristic?"
- **Apply the same risk-based rigor to service and field tools** Any tool verifying a safety-critical characteristic — anywhere in the lifecycle — belongs in the risk-based tier.

Measurement is the mechanism by which risk controls are confirmed to exist in the product as it reaches the patient. When the measurement system is not calibrated appropriately for the task it performs, the confirmation is unreliable — and ultimately, patient safety is compromised.

Notes & Sources

- **On the obligation to assess previous measurement results when equipment is found out of calibration** — ISO 13485:2016, Clause 7.6.

Chapter 20: Supplier Engineering & Supplier Quality

Medical device manufacturers source components, materials, sub-assemblies, and services from hundreds of suppliers. In large organizations, the supply chain touches nearly every element of the finished device — raw materials, molded and machined parts, electronic assemblies, software, sterilization, packaging, calibration services, and more. Managing this supply chain is a significant operational undertaking. Supplier quality is responsible for ensuring that incoming parts meet requirements, that suppliers remain capable, and that the supply chain does not introduce risks that compromise patient safety.

This chapter focuses on the specific places where supplier quality decisions intersect with the product risk management file — and what those decisions look like when **patient safety** is the governing question.

The Responsibility That Cannot Be Delegated

Before discussing specific activities, one foundational principle must be stated clearly because everything else depends on it.

No supplier certification, no quality agreement, no audit record, and no certificate of conformance transfers the manufacturer's responsibility for patient safety. A supplier can perform work, produce components, and hold certifications. But if a patient is harmed by a device containing a defective component from a qualified supplier, the responsibility remains with the manufacturer — because **responsibility for patient safety cannot be outsourced**.

This is the operating premise behind every risk-based supplier decision. When a supplier engineer asks, *"How much oversight does this supplier need?"* the underlying question is: How much patient safety risk are we accepting if this supplier produces a nonconforming component and we do not detect it?

The answer lies in the risk management file. Supplier engineers who understand this approach make oversight decisions differently — because they know what the component actually does for the patient.

Component Criticality: What the Risk Management File Tells You Before Anything Else

The first patient safety connection in supplier quality occurs before any supplier is contacted, before qualification begins, and before incoming inspection is designed. It begins with a simple question:

Which components and materials are safety-critical?

The hazard analysis identifies device characteristics whose acceptable ranges are defined because deviation contributes to a hazardous situation. Any component or material that implements or directly affects one of these characteristics is a **safety-critical component**. Any supplier producing such a component is a **safety-critical supplier**.

This seems obvious when stated plainly. In practice, it is rarely formalized. Supplier classification systems often rely on generic criteria — custom vs. off-the-shelf, sole-source vs. multi-source, special handling vs. standard — without explicitly tracing to the product risk management file. A component may be labeled "standard" in the supplier management system while corresponding to a high-severity hazardous situation in the risk file. The supplier engineer may never know the discrepancy exists.

Why this matters: A supplier classification system that does not reflect the device's risk cannot be risk-based — and cannot protect patients.

The risk-based consideration at this stage is straightforward: Run the component list against the hazard analysis. For each component, ask: does this component implement a risk control or contribute to a hazardous situation? At what risk level?

These answers form the foundation for every downstream supplier decision — qualification rigor, quality agreement depth, incoming inspection strategy, and SCAR urgency.

This mapping must be updated whenever the risk management file changes — when new risks are characterized, when risk controls are modified, or when severity assessments shift. A supplier program built on outdated assumptions about component criticality is a program built on flawed information.

Supplier Selection and Qualification: Matching Rigor to Stakes

Supplier qualification determines whether a supplier can reliably produce parts that meet the manufacturer's needs. For safety-critical parts, the question becomes: Is the supplier capable of consistently producing the safety-critical attributes that the device relies on?

A generic supplier audit may confirm that the supplier has documentation, trained personnel, calibrated equipment, and an active CAPA system. These are necessary — but insufficient — for safety-critical components. The manufacturer must also ensure that the supplier can produce the **specific critical attributes**: material composition, tolerance levels, surface properties, mechanical strength, or any characteristic tied to a risk control.

Contract Manufacturers (CMOs): The Highest Stakes

Among all suppliers, contract manufacturers carry the greatest responsibility. Every control measure in the risk management file ultimately passes through the manufacturing process. Outsourcing production does not outsource responsibility for patient safety — it only delegates the actions necessary to ensure it.

Qualification of a CMO must therefore include:

- evaluation of the supplier's overall QMS,
- verification of capability to perform safety-critical process steps,
- confirmation that process validation exists and remains valid,

- and assurance that changes affecting safety-critical characteristics cannot occur without notification.

Quality Agreements: Extending Risk Management Into the Supply Chain

Quality agreements are the contractual mechanism through which the manufacturer extends its risk management framework to suppliers. For safety-critical suppliers, quality agreements must:

- define what constitutes a significant change requiring notification,
- specify audit rights (including unannounced access when appropriate),
- require maintenance of process validation for safety-critical processes,
- and mandate flow-down of controls to sub-tier suppliers.

Quality agreements for commodity suppliers — those providing non-critical components — do not require this depth. Applying the same template to all suppliers creates administrative burden without adding patient safety value. Differentiating agreement depth based on component criticality is itself a **risk-based decision**, and the risk management file makes that differentiation defensible.

Incoming Inspection: The Last Internal Defense

Every component entering the facility is either verified through inspection or accepted based on supplier certification and historical performance. Incoming inspection strategy — how much verification to perform and for which characteristics — is a risk-based decision that many organizations make without reference to the risk management file.

ISO 13485:2016, Clause 7.4.3, makes the connection explicit: the extent of verification must be based on supplier evaluation and the risk to the final product.

For safety-critical components, incoming inspection must answer: Does this lot contain the safety-critical characteristic within its acceptable range? This may require direct measurement, not just acceptance of a certificate of conformance.

Accepting a safety-critical component on certificate alone is a **risk acceptance decision**. It assumes:

- the supplier's measurement system is reliable,
- the process producing the characteristic has not changed,
- and any deviation would have been detected and disclosed.

For a supplier with a long, stable history of capability, this may be acceptable. For a newer supplier, one with recent nonconformances, or one without strong change-notification obligations, it may not be.

When incoming inspection includes physical verification of safety-critical characteristics, the sampling plan must be **commensurate with the safety risk** if a nonconforming component reaches a patient. Higher severity requires more rigorous verification.

Why this matters: Incoming inspection is the last point at which a nonconforming safety-critical component can be detected before it enters production — and potentially reaches a patient. The cost of being wrong is direct patient harm.

SCARs: Urgency and Depth Proportionate to Patient Safety Stakes

When a supplier produces a nonconforming component — discovered at incoming inspection, during manufacturing, through complaints, or via audit — the manufacturer must decide whether to issue a Supplier Corrective Action Request (SCAR). That decision, and everything that follows if a SCAR is issued, should be governed by the same principle that governs every other risk-based decision: the severity of patient harm if the nonconformance reaches a patient in a finished device

For non-critical components (cosmetic defects, non-functional dimensional deviations), SCAR urgency and depth are proportionate to quality impact.

For safety-critical components, a SCAR is a **patient safety response**. Treating these situations with the same urgency and investigation depth as cosmetic issues has made a risk acceptance decision without recognizing it: they have accepted the patient safety risk of a slow or shallow response to a safety-critical supplier problem.

Risk-based decisions in a SCAR include:

1. **Should a SCAR be issued?** For safety-critical components, the threshold is lower. A first-occurrence nonconformance in a safety-critical attribute warrants a SCAR.
2. **What response timeline is required?** Timelines must be commensurate with severity. A component tied to a catastrophic hazard requires a more urgent response than one tied to moderate severity.
3. **What depth of investigation is adequate?** For safety-critical failures, corrective action must address the **systemic root cause**, not just the symptom.
4. **How should effectiveness be verified?** Effectiveness must confirm that the **risk of recurrence** — and thus the risk to patients — has been reduced to an acceptable level.

Additional Risks the Device Risk Management File Should Know About

Sub-tier Supplier Changes

A quality agreement with a tier-1 supplier does not guarantee control over tier-2 suppliers.

Example: A resin formulation change at a sub-tier supplier — communicated to the tier-1 supplier but not to the manufacturer — can alter safety-critical attributes without detection. Quality agreements for safety-critical components must require sub-tier change notification, even if enforcement is challenging.

Component Obsolescence

When a safety-critical component is discontinued, replacement qualification must evaluate the safety-critical characteristic directly — not assume equivalence based on dimensions or product family or same-supplier-sourcing. A "like-for-like" substitution that bypasses safety-critical testing invalidates assumptions in the risk management file.

What Risk Management Actually Needs from You

Risk management needs supplier engineers to:

- **Classify components based on the potential risk of failure and the risk controls they implement** Supplier criticality must trace to the hazard analysis, not generic criteria.
- **Match qualification rigor to patient safety stakes** Safety-critical suppliers — especially CMOs — require deeper evaluation and stronger controls.
- **Design quality agreements that reflect component criticality** Change notification, audit rights, and flow-down obligations must be **commensurate with risk**.

- **Set incoming inspection strategies based on severity** Sampling plans and acceptance criteria must reflect the harm that could occur if a nonconforming component reaches a patient.
- **Escalate SCARs with urgency proportionate to patient safety impact** Safety-critical failures require faster timelines, deeper investigations, and stronger corrective actions.
- **Capture sub-tier and obsolescence risks in the risk management file** Lifecycle changes must be reassessed for their impact on safety-critical characteristics.

And every supplier quality engineer — from entry-level to experienced — must internalize the principle that opened this chapter: **the manufacturer's responsibility for patient safety cannot be delegated.** The risk management file is the document that tells the supplier quality function what that responsibility requires, component by component, decision by decision.

Notes & Sources

- **On risk-based supplier classification and incoming inspection extent** — ISO 13485:2016, Clauses 7.4.1 and 7.4.3.

Part IV — Regulatory, Clinical & Market Access Functions

Chapter 21: Regulatory Affairs

Classification and Pathway: A Risk Acceptance Decision

Device classification is the regulatory system's risk-based determination of how much evidence is required before a device can be used on patients. In the United States, FDA classifies devices into three categories:

- **Class I** devices are subject to general controls, which are considered sufficient to ensure safety and effectiveness.
- **Class II** devices require special controls, often demonstrated through a **510(k)** submission showing *substantial equivalence* to a legally marketed predicate.
- **Class III** devices require premarket approval (PMA) supported by valid scientific evidence, typically including clinical data.

Under EU MDR Annex VIII, devices are classified as **Class I, IIa, IIb, or III** based on intended use, invasiveness, duration of contact, and other risk-relevant factors. Higher classes require Notified Body involvement and more rigorous conformity assessment.

Why this matters: Classification sets the evidence ceiling. Before a single test is run or a single patient is enrolled, classification determines how much safety evidence must be generated. A device classified lower than its true risk profile results in an evidence obligation below the level commensurate with patient safety risk.

Therefore, classification must be grounded in the device's actual risk profile — not in predicate availability, pathway speed, or commercial timelines. The risk management file's characterization of hazards and severity is the evidence that should inform the classification judgment.

A device whose hazard analysis identifies multiple high-severity or catastrophic hazardous situations — especially those requiring complex risk controls whose effectiveness has not been demonstrated clinically — has a risk profile that warrants careful consideration of whether the proposed pathway's evidence requirements are adequate.

Predicate Selection: A Safety Decision, Not a Procedural One

Predicate selection in a 510(k) submission also carries a patient safety dimension. Substantial equivalence requires demonstrating:

- the same intended use, and
- technological characteristics that do not raise new safety concerns.

Whether new technological features raise new safety concerns is itself a **risk assessment**. It requires asking:

- Do the new technological characteristics introduce hazards the predicate did not?
- Does the evidence package address those hazards?
- Does the risk management file reflect the differences accurately?

A predicate chosen for convenience rather than safety alignment creates a weak safety argument — and reviewers will find the gap.

The Submission As an Evidence Argument, not a Documentation Exercise

When preparing a regulatory submission — whether a 510(k), PMA, De Novo, or EU MDR Technical Documentation — the **risk management file becomes the core of the evidence**. It is where the manufacturer demonstrates:

- the risks associated with the device,
- the severity and probability of those risks,
- the risk controls implemented,
- the verification of those controls, and
- the residual risk and benefit–risk conclusion.

Regulatory affairs is not responsible for compiling the risk management file, but it **is** responsible for evaluating it as a reviewer would. The question is not "Is the file complete?" but:

Does this file answer the questions a competent regulator or Notified Body will ask?

Examples of credibility gaps include:

- A risk management file assigning severity levels inconsistent with clinical literature for the patient population.
- Risk controls that are not verified through design verification or clinical evidence.
- Residual risk conclusions that do not align with the device's intended use or known clinical risks.

Why this matters: A submission that assembles documents without a coherent safety argument forces the reviewer to build that argument themselves — and they will do so more conservatively than the manufacturer would.

FDA and ISO 14971: A Direct Regulatory Bridge

FDA's recognition of **ISO 14971:2019** as a consensus standard creates a direct bridge between the manufacturer's risk management file and FDA's safety expectations. When a manufacturer cites ISO 14971 in a submission, FDA reviewers and investigators expect the file to reflect the standard's requirements.

Gaps between ISO 14971 and the actual file are not documentation issues — **they are patient safety findings**.

EU MDR: Risk Management as a Legal Obligation

Under EU MDR, the requirement is even more explicit. Annex I, Section 3 mandates that manufacturers establish, implement, document, and maintain a risk management system. The General Safety and Performance Requirements (GSPR) require:

- all known and foreseeable risks to be minimized,
- risks to be acceptable relative to clinical benefits,
- a continuous, iterative risk management process throughout the lifecycle, and
- evidence linking each GSPR requirement to objective proof.

For GSPR Sections 1–9, this evidence is primarily the **risk management output**.

Regulatory affairs must therefore ask:

- Does the intended use statement match the hazard analysis?
- Are harms defined at severity levels consistent with clinical evidence?
- Are risk mitigations implemented and demonstrably effective?
- Is the benefit–risk conclusion aligned with residual risks?

The regulatory affairs professional who asks these questions before submission is the last internal safeguard between a weak safety argument and the reviewer who will identify the gap.

Post-Market Changes: The Submission Trigger Is a Risk Management Question

Once a device is on the market, regulatory affairs must determine whether changes — design updates, software modifications, manufacturing changes, labeling revisions — require a new submission or can be handled internally. This is one of the most frequent and consequential patient safety decisions regulatory affairs makes.

FDA: 21 CFR 807.81(a)(3)

A new 510(k) is required when a change **could significantly affect safety or effectiveness**. FDA guidance provides flowcharts and decision trees for evaluating:

- intended use changes,
- design changes,
- material changes,
- software changes,
- manufacturing changes.

These tools are useful — but insufficient on their own. The key question in every flowchart branch is: **Does this change significantly affect safety or effectiveness?**

That is a **risk management question**, and it cannot be answered without referencing the risk management file.

For example: A software change that modifies a timing parameter may not trigger any explicit flowchart thresholds. But if that timing parameter governs a safety-critical alarm — if it implements a risk control for a high-severity hazard — then the change may significantly affect safety even if the flowchart does not surface it. Only the risk management file reveals this connection.

EU MDR: Conformity and GSPR Impact

Under EU MDR, changes must be assessed for their impact on conformity with the GSPR and the Technical Documentation. Any change that affects:

- the risk management file's conclusions,
- the implementation of risk controls, or
- the benefit–risk characterization,

requires Notified Body notification and may require supplementary assessment.

Where FDA provides explicit flowcharts, EU MDR emphasizes **documented justification** that the change's impact on conformity has been fully assessed. Both systems require the same underlying step: **review the risk management file**.

Why this matters: A submission trigger determination made without reading the risk management file is a determination made without the most important information about whether the change matters for patient safety.

Regulatory affairs professionals who embed a mandatory risk management file review into change assessment make defensible decisions — because they are grounded in evidence about what the change means for the patient.

What Risk Management Actually Needs from You

Risk management needs regulatory affairs professionals to:

- **Treat classification and pathway selection as patient safety decisions.** Evidence obligations must be **commensurate with the device's true risk profile**, not commercial convenience.

- **Evaluate the risk management file as the core of the safety argument.** Regulators read it as evidence of whether the manufacturer understands the risks of its own device.
- **Ensure the submission tells a coherent safety story.** The risk management file must align with clinical evidence, verification data, and intended use.
- **Use the risk management file to evaluate predicate selection.** Differences in technological characteristics must be assessed for new hazards.
- **Ground post-market change assessments in risk management.** Every change must be evaluated for its impact on risk controls, hazardous situations, and benefit–risk conclusions.
- **Recognize that regulatory affairs is the final internal reviewer.** The regulatory submission is the manufacturer's patient safety argument. The risk management file *is* that argument.

The regulatory affairs professional who owns the quality of that argument — who asks whether the evidence truly supports the claims being made — is doing work that matters directly for patient safety.

Chapter 22: Medical Affairs & Clinical Evidence

Severity of harm is a clinical judgment. It asks: **if a patient in the target population is exposed to this hazardous situation, what actually happens to them?** Does their condition deteriorate reversibly or irreversibly? Is the harm detectable in time for intervention? Does the patient's underlying disease make them more or less vulnerable? Is the harm an inconvenience, a complication, a permanent injury, or a death?

These questions cannot be answered by reading a device specification. They require understanding the **clinical context** — the patient, the disease, the standard of care, and the consequences of intervention failure. The people in a medical device organization who hold this knowledge are the medical affairs professionals, clinical scientists, and medically trained reviewers whose job is to understand and curate clinical evidence.

A similar principle applies to **benefit** in the benefit–risk equation. Every risk management file that performs a benefit–risk analysis must characterize the clinical benefit against which residual risk is weighed: how much the device reduces mortality, how meaningfully it improves function, how it compares to available alternatives, and what the patient's clinical course would be without it. These are clinical questions, and they require clinical expertise.

This chapter addresses the specific places where medical affairs professionals contribute clinical expertise to the risk management file — and what those contributions look like when they are made deliberately rather than incidentally.

Severity Is a Clinical Judgment, not Merely a Scale Selection

ISO 14971 requires that the severity of harm be estimated for each identified hazardous situation. The standard is explicit that this estimate must reflect the **nature of the harm** —

reversible or irreversible, temporary or permanent, minor or catastrophic — and the **clinical context** of the patient population exposed to it. What the standard does not specify is **who** should make this estimate, leaving many organizations to assign it to whoever is building the risk management file.

The result is predictable: severity is often estimated from the device's perspective rather than the patient's.

For example:

- A **delayed alarm** is labeled "moderate severity" because the delay is brief by engineering standards — without asking what a brief delay means for a patient in **septic shock**, where irreversible deterioration can occur within minutes.
- A **drug dose misinterpretation** is labeled "negligible" because the numerical difference seems small — without considering whether even a small dosing error could cause severe harm from overdose or underdose.
- A **momentary loss of pacing** in a cardiac device is labeled "temporary" because the interruption is short — without considering that in certain arrhythmias, even seconds of lost pacing can be life-threatening.

These are not hypothetical. They represent the failure pattern that clinical review consistently uncovers in engineering-led severity estimates.

Medical affairs professionals — medical directors, clinical scientists, physicians with therapeutic expertise — are best positioned to ground severity estimates in clinical reality. Their contribution is not to override engineering understanding of how the device fails, but to analyze the **clinical consequence** of each hazardous situation: **Given this patient population, this clinical setting, and this underlying condition, what actually happens to the patient when this hazardous situation occurs?**

A risk management file whose severity estimates have been reviewed and confirmed by clinical experts ensures that downstream decisions — what requires risk reduction, what requires benefit–risk justification, what can be accepted — are **commensurate with the true clinical consequences**, not engineering convention.

Why this matters: Severity drives everything downstream: risk control priority, benefit–risk justification, and ultimately whether the device is safe enough for patients. If severity is wrong, everything built on top of it is wrong.

Probability Estimation: Where Clinical Literature Meets the Hazard Analysis

ISO 14971 decomposes the probability of harm into two components:

- **P1** — the probability that a hazardous situation occurs
- **P2** — the probability that the hazardous situation leads to harm

P1 is largely a device and process question. P2 is a **clinical** question.

P2 depends on:

- whether clinical intervention is available and effective,
- how rapidly the patient's condition deteriorates once exposed,
- whether age, comorbidities, or disease severity increase vulnerability,
- whether the clinical setting (ICU vs. home use) affects detectability or response time.

These factors are not found in device specifications or failure mode analyses. They are found in: clinical literature, registry data, adverse event databases for comparable devices, and the clinical experience of practitioners. For example:

- Literature may show that **untreated ventricular arrhythmias** lead to death in 60% of cases within minutes — a direct input to P2 for hazardous situations involving delayed arrhythmia detection.
- Registry data may show that **catheter occlusions** in certain patient groups lead to sepsis in 20–30% of cases — a direct input to P2 for occlusion-related hazards.
- Clinical studies may show that **missed hypoglycemia alarms** in pediatric patients lead to severe harm far more frequently than in adults — a population-specific P2 adjustment.

The literature review conducted for clinical evaluation often contains incidence rates for complications, intervention success rates, and data on the clinical course of the underlying condition. This is **probability data**, and it should flow directly into the risk management file's P2 estimates.

In most organizations, this connection does not exist. Clinical literature lives in one system; hazard analysis lives in another. Probability estimates are assigned using internal scales without systematic reference to the clinical evidence medical affairs has already compiled.

Why this matters: If P2 is underestimated, the risk score is artificially low — and risk controls may not be implemented where they are needed.

The integration that serves patient safety is simple: Medical affairs should identify the clinical evidence most relevant to P2 and use it to explicitly inform the risk management file.

Clinical Evidence at Development: Grounding the Risk Management File Before Market Launch

Before a device reaches its first patient outside a controlled study, the risk management file contains risk estimates, risk controls, and a benefit–risk conclusion based on **pre-market evidence**. The quality of that evidence — its relevance, completeness, and honesty about limitations — determines the strength of the benefit–risk conclusion.

Medical affairs contributes to this evidence base in two primary ways.

1. State-of-the-Art Analysis

ISO 14971 requires that risk management consider the **state of the art** — the current clinical and technical standards used to evaluate performance and safety. MEDDEV 2.7/1 Rev. 4 requires that clinical evaluation establish:

- the current standard of care,
- the risks and benefits of available alternatives,
- and the clinical need the device addresses.

This analysis becomes the reference point against which the benefit–risk conclusion is judged:

Is the device's benefit–risk profile at least equivalent to, and ideally better than, the alternatives available to the patient?

2. Pre-Market Clinical Study Design and Interpretation

Where clinical investigations are conducted, the data they generate are the most direct pre-market evidence for both probability estimation and benefit quantification.

Medical affairs professionals designing and interpreting these studies must ensure:

- the endpoints address safety-critical risks,
- the patient population reflects real-world use,
- the follow-up period is long enough to detect clinically meaningful harms,
- and the study evaluates the risks the risk management file identifies as most consequential.

A study designed only to satisfy regulatory requirements may not generate the evidence needed to support a robust benefit–risk conclusion.

Why this matters: Pre-market evidence sets the **initial hypothesis** about benefit–risk. Chapter 23 will address what happens when post-market evidence proves that hypothesis true.

Benefit-Risk Analysis: The Clinical Argument the Risk Management File Must Make

ISO 14971:2019 requires a benefit–risk analysis when residual risks exceed acceptance criteria. EU MDR Annex I, Section 8 requires that all known and foreseeable risks be reduced **as far as possible** and be acceptable relative to clinical benefits. This is a **continuous** obligation, not a one-time pre-market exercise.

The benefit–risk analysis is where clinical evidence must appear explicitly. Also, FDA's benefit–risk guidance identifies the benefit factors that should inform this analysis:

- **Type of benefit** — impact on treatment, function, or quality of life
- **Magnitude of benefit** — measurable clinical improvement
- **Probability of benefit** — likelihood the patient will experience it
- **Duration of benefit** — how long the benefit lasts
- **Patient perspective** — how patients value the benefit relative to risks

Each of these requires clinical evidence and clinical interpretation. For example:

- Magnitude of benefit requires comparing outcomes **with and without** the device.

- Probability of benefit requires evidence of device performance in the **actual patient population.**
- Duration of benefit requires **follow-up data** from studies or real-world use.

Medical affairs professionals hold this evidence. They conduct systematic literature reviews, interpret clinical study results, and maintain awareness of evolving clinical data.

Why this matters: A benefit–risk analysis without clinical evidence is not an analysis — it is an assumption.

What Risk Management Actually Needs from You

Risk management needs medical affairs professionals to:

- **Ground severity estimates in clinical reality** Severity must reflect what actually happens to patients — not engineering intuition.
- **Provide clinical evidence for P2 probability estimates.** Literature, registries, and clinical experience must inform how likely harm is once a hazardous situation occurs.
- **Ensure benefit characterization is evidence-based.** Magnitude, likelihood, and duration of benefit must be supported by clinical data.
- **Define the state of the art and clinical context.** Risk management decisions must be made relative to current clinical practice and available alternatives.
- **Shape pre-market clinical studies to address safety-critical risks.** Study design must be aligned with the risk profile, not just regulatory minimums.
- **Maintain clinical coherence across the risk management file.** Severity, probability, and benefit

must be **commensurate with the clinical consequences** for the patient.

Medical affairs provides the clinical truth that anchors the risk management file in patient reality. Without that truth, the file becomes an engineering document — not a safety document.

Notes & Sources

- **On benefit-risk analysis and the clinical evidence required to conduct it** — FDA, "Factors to Consider Regarding Benefit-Risk," 2019; ISO/TR 24971:2020; ISO 14971:2019.
- **On state-of-the-art analysis as a risk management input** — MEDDEV 2.7/1 Rev 4, Sections 7 and 8.
- **On clinical investigation standards for pre-market and post-market clinical studies** — ISO 14155:2020.

Chapter 23: Clinical Safety, Vigilance & Post-Market Clinical Follow-Up (PMCF)

When a medical device reaches the market, the risk management file reflects the manufacturer's **best pre-market assessment** of hazards, risks, risk controls, and the benefit–risk balance. That assessment is built on pre-market evidence — bench testing, clinical studies, literature reviews, engineering analyses. It represents what was known **before** any patient outside a controlled study used the device in real clinical practice.

Once the device enters the real world, the question becomes: **Does reality still match what the risk management file predicted?**

This chapter addresses the full clinical safety and vigilance lifecycle — adverse event evaluation, vigilance reporting, and the post-market clinical evidence frameworks that govern how real-world data feeds back into the risk management file. EU MDR's structured requirements and FDA's parallel expectations are addressed at each stage.

Adverse Event Evaluation

Adverse event evaluation is a **risk-based decision** at its core. It requires determining whether the reported incident corresponds to a hazardous situation characterized in the risk management file — and if so, what the event reveals about the **probability and severity assumptions** made during pre-market assessment.

This distinction matters because **regulatory reporting thresholds and risk-management thresholds are not the same**.

An event may be **below the regulatory reporting threshold** — not a "serious incident" under EU MDR or not reportable under FDA MDR — yet still provide evidence that the device's **risk profile needs re-evaluation**.

For example:

- A series of **non-serious occlusion alarms** in an infusion pump may not trigger vigilance reporting but may indicate that the real-world probability of occlusion is higher than estimated.
- Repeated **minor skin injuries** from a wearable device may not be reportable individually but may reveal a pattern of harm in a vulnerable subpopulation (e.g., elderly patients with fragile skin).

The most important risk-based decision the clinical safety professional makes is not whether any single event is reportable. It is whether the **pattern of events** is consistent with the risk management file's assumptions — and whether the accumulating data is telling the organization something new about its device in real-world use.

Why this matters: If adverse event patterns diverge from the risk file's assumptions, the device's safety case is no longer accurate — and patient safety decisions become misaligned with reality.

Vigilance Reporting: The Regulatory Obligation Grounded in Risk

Medical device vigilance — the formal system for reporting serious incidents, field safety corrective actions (FSCAs), and trends in non-serious incidents is the manufacturer's ongoing patient safety monitoring. The vigilance report is a regulatory document, but the **decision to file it is a risk-based judgment**.

Under EU MDR:

- **Serious incidents** must be reported.
- Each serious incident must be evaluated for its implications for **FSCA obligations**.

The threshold is explicitly risk-based: **Does the event or pattern of events indicate that the device's residual risk has become unacceptable in light of new information?**

This determination requires referencing the **residual risk characterization** in the risk management file and evaluating whether field data is consistent with the assumptions underlying that characterization.

FDA does not have an FSCA framework identical to EU MDR, but **corrections and removals** under 21 CFR Part 806 apply when an action is taken to reduce a health risk. This is further discussed in Chapter 28. This determination requires the same risk-based reasoning: **Does the event indicate that the device's risk is greater than previously understood?**

Why this matters: Vigilance reporting is not a paperwork exercise. It is a **patient safety decision** grounded in whether the device's real-world performance remains consistent with the risk the manufacturer judged acceptable at market entry.

The EU MDR Post-Market Clinical Evidence Framework: PMCF, CER, PSUR, and the Living Risk Management File

EU MDR introduces a structured, mandatory post-market clinical evidence system. Understanding how each component connects to the risk management file is essential.

Post-Market Clinical Follow-Up (PMCF): PMCF, defined in Annex XIV Part B, is an **ongoing, proactive procedure** for gathering and assessing clinical data from real-world use. PMCF is **not optional**. Every manufacturer must have a PMCF plan, regardless of device class.

The scope and depth of PMCF must be **commensurate with device risk**. For example, a Class III cardiac implant requires intensive, targeted PMCF. A Class I wound dressing requires proportionate but still structured PMCF.

PMCF aims to:

- confirm long-term safety and performance,

- monitor the ongoing acceptability of identified risks,
- identify new risks not apparent pre-market,
- ensure the benefit–risk balance remains acceptable.

PMCF Integration to Patient Safety: All PMCF activities — registry studies, prospective studies, literature reviews, user surveys — generate evidence that must be assessed for implications to the risk management file.

Examples:

- A registry showing **higher-than-expected stroke rates** for a vascular device requires re-evaluation of P2 and benefit–risk.
- A user survey revealing **unexpected usability challenges** may indicate a hazardous situation not previously characterized.
- Literature showing **new contraindications** for a patient subgroup may require updating severity or probability estimates.

The PMCF Evaluation Report feeds directly into the **CER update**, which must remain consistent with the risk management file.

Clinical Evaluation Report (CER): The CER, required under Annex XIV Part A and Article 61, is a **living document.** It must be updated **annually** for Class III and implantable devices, and **every two years** for Class IIb devices.

Each update must ensure that the **residual risk categorization** in the risk management file aligns with the CER's benefit–risk conclusion.

Periodic Safety Update Report (PSUR): PSURs, required under **Article 86**, apply to Class IIa, IIb, and III devices. They must include:

- a summary of post-market data,
- a revised benefit–risk determination,
- conclusions on corrective or preventive actions.

Class IIb and III devices require **annual** PSURs.

Post-Market Surveillance Report (PMSR): PMSRs, required under **Article 85**, apply to Class I devices. They are lighter than PSURs but serve the same purpose: ensuring systematic review of post-market data and its implications for safety.

The architecture governed by EU MDR is therefore a continuous feedback loop: **PMCF → PMCF Evaluation Report → CER Update → PSUR/PMSR → Risk Management File**

At every point, the risk management file is the **core reference**.

Why this matters: EU MDR mandates the architecture — but only the manufacturer can ensure the loop actually closes. Documents can exist in parallel without ever informing each other unless the organization deliberately integrates them.

The FDA Parallel

FDA does not require PMCF, CER, PSUR, or PMSR. Instead, post-market clinical evidence obligations appear through:

- **Post-approval studies** for PMA devices,
- **Post-market surveillance studies** under 21 CFR Part 822 for certain Class II and III devices,
- **ISO 14971:2019 Clause 10**, requiring systematic review of production and post-production information.

The patient safety obligation is the same: **real-world evidence must feed back into the risk management file.**

The difference is structural:

- Under EU MDR, the architecture is mandated.
- Under FDA, the manufacturer must build the architecture deliberately.

Why this matters: Manufacturers operating under FDA must create the feedback loop intentionally. Manufacturers under EU MDR must ensure the mandated loop is actually functional — not just documented.

Risk-Based Decisions in Clinical Safety and Vigilance: What the Risk Management File Governs

The clinical safety and vigilance function makes several recurring risk-based decisions. Each is correct only when the risk management file is the governing reference.

1. Does this pattern of adverse events indicate that the probability estimate is wrong?

Trending complaints against risk management file characterizations — when proceduralized — becomes an early warning system for product risk.

2. Does this PMCF finding change the benefit–risk conclusion?

PMCF data showing higher-than-expected adverse event rates, or more vulnerable patient populations, or lower-than-expected benefits, requires re-evaluation of the benefit–risk conclusion.

3. Should a field safety corrective action (FSCA) be initiated?

Under EU MDR, this determination is explicitly tied to the risk management file: **Does the field data indicate that the device's residual risk has become unacceptable?**

Under FDA, the same substantive question is asked through the corrections and removals framework.

Why this matters: Every post-market safety decision is, at its core, a question about whether the device's real-world performance still matches the risk that the manufacturer judged acceptable at market entry.

What Risk Management Actually Needs from You

Risk management needs clinical safety and vigilance professionals to:

- **Evaluate every adverse event as a query against the risk management file.** Does the event align with the predicted hazardous situations, severity, and probability?
- **Trend events, not just classify them.** Patterns of non-serious events may reveal probability shifts before serious incidents occur.
- **Integrate PMCF findings into risk re-evaluation.** PMCF evidence must inform updates to severity, probability, and benefit–risk conclusions.
- **Use the risk management file to guide FSCA decisions.** The threshold for action is whether residual risk has become unacceptable.
- **Ensure post-market evidence is commensurate with device risk.** Higher-risk devices require deeper, more frequent, and more structured evidence collection.
- **Maintain the living nature of the risk management file.** Real-world evidence must continuously update the file so that it reflects patient reality, not pre-market assumptions.

Patients need assurance that the manufacturer understands how acceptable the device's risks truly are. That understanding lives in the risk management file — and clinical safety provides the real-world evidence that keeps it honest.

Notes & Sources

- **On the EU MDR serious incident reporting obligations and vigilance framework** — EU MDR 2017/745, Articles 83, 87–92.
- **On FDA adverse event reporting and corrections and removals** — 21 CFR Part 803; 21 CFR Part 806.

Chapter 24: Labeling, IFU & User Training

The IFU Is a Risk Control Measure

Instructions for Use (IFU), device labeling, quick reference guides, and technical manuals are not incidental add-ons to a medical device. They are structural components of the device's design and **risk control architecture**.

ISO 14971 establishes a hierarchy of risk control options. When a hazard is identified and the associated risk is unacceptable, the manufacturer must:

1. **First**, attempt to reduce the risk through **inherent safe design** — eliminating the hazardous situation.
2. **Second**, implement **protective measures** — guards, interlocks, alarms, automatic shutoffs.
3. **Only third**, when design and protective measures cannot fully reduce risk, provide **information for safety** — instructions, warnings, cautions, contraindications, and training.

This hierarchy means something profound: **Every safety-related statement in the IFU is a risk control measure.**

ISO 20417 makes this explicit by requiring that labeling content integrate with ISO 14971 risk management principles. Safety-critical information identified through the risk management process must be communicated in labeling in a way that supports safe and effective device use.

The practical consequence is clear: **Every warning, caution, contraindication, and limitation in the IFU must be traceable to a specific residual risk in the risk management file.**

If a warning exists without a corresponding residual risk, the risk management file is incomplete — or the warning is unnecessary. If a residual risk requires user communication but has no corresponding IFU statement, the risk control is documented but not implemented.

Both are patient safety gaps.

The labeling engineer who reviews the IFU against the risk management file is performing a traceability review that many organizations conduct only at submission time — if at all.

Why this matters: Labeling is not a compliance artifact. It is the final implementation of many risk controls. If labeling is wrong, incomplete, or misaligned with the risk file, the device's safety architecture collapses at the point closest to the patient.

Risk-Based Categorization: Warnings, Cautions, Contraindications, Limitations

Under EU MDR Annex I, Section 23, information supplied by the manufacturer — labels, IFU, and accompanying documentation — is a legal requirement for CE marking. Residual risks of clinical significance must be disclosed, and information must be sufficient to allow safe use. FDA's 21 CFR Part 801 requires labeling to be truthful, not misleading, and to include adequate directions for use.

Within this regulatory framework, categorization decisions in the IFU are risk-based decisions:

- Warnings communicate conditions requiring specific user action to prevent or reduce harm.
- Cautions communicate conditions requiring attention to avoid less severe consequences.
- Contraindications communicate situations where the device should not be used because the risk exceeds the benefit for a specific patient population.
- Limitations communicate constraints on device use that represent residual risks the manufacturer cannot further reduce.

ISO/TR 24971 Annex D provides guidance on these categories, and ISO 20417 implements them in IFU structure.

A labeling engineer who categorizes a catastrophic-severity residual risk as a caution has made a categorization error with direct patient safety implications. Conversely, labeling a minor residual risk as a warning dilutes the prominence of truly critical warnings.

Why this matters: The prominence, placement, and categorization of safety information must be commensurate with the severity of harm it is intended to prevent. Misclassification is not a formatting error — it is a patient safety error.

Information for Safety vs. Residual Risk Disclosure: The Most Consequential Distinction in Labeling

ISO 14971 and ISO/TR 24971 draw a distinction that is simple in concept but consistently misunderstood in practice:

Information for Safety = Risk Control

Information for safety instructs the user on what to do — or not do — to avoid a hazardous situation or reduce its likelihood or severity. Examples:

- "Before connecting the patient cable, verify that the grounding lead is securely attached."
- "Do not use this device on patients with implanted electronic stimulation devices."
- "After each use, inspect the connector for visible damage before storing."

If followed, these statements **reduce risk**. Therefore, they must be **verified for effectiveness**. And verification is not a documentation review. It is a **human performance test**:

- Do intended users read the statement?
- Do they understand it?

- Do they perform the required action correctly under realistic conditions?

IEC 62366 and FDA's Human Factors guidance provide the framework for this verification. This is discussed in detail in Chapter 10.

Residual Risk Disclosure = Transparency, Not Control

Residual risk disclosure informs users that a risk remains despite risk controls. Examples:

- "Patients may experience temporary discomfort at the application site."
- "There is a small risk of infection associated with any invasive procedure."

These statements do **not** reduce risk. They acknowledge it.

ISO/TR 24971 is clear: residual risk disclosure is not a risk control measure.

Why this matters: Confusing these categories leads to two dangerous outcomes.

1. **Over-reliance on labeling** as the primary control for high-severity hazards.
2. **Under-communication** of clinically significant residual risks.

Information for safety is the weakest risk control in the hierarchy for a reason: its effectiveness depends on user literacy, cognitive load, and environmental conditions the manufacturer cannot control.

A labeling team that writes warnings for catastrophic hazards must ask the critical question: **Why is this being handled in the IFU rather than in the design?**

Foreseeable Misuse Flows Both Ways

Most organizations treat the relationship between the risk management file and the IFU as one-directional: risk management outputs → labeling inputs.

But the relationship is **bidirectional**. ISO 14971 requires hazard analysis to consider both intended use and **reasonably foreseeable misuse**. IEC 62366 explicitly includes labeling and IFU content as part of the user interface whose usability studies determine which use errors are foreseeable.

For example: A summative usability evaluation reveals that **30% of test participants** attempt to use the device on a contraindicated patient type because they misread the contraindication section. This is a foreseeable misuse scenario that must be assessed in the hazard analysis.

The risk management team cannot identify this hazard without the labeling team's insight into how the IFU actually functions in users' hands.

When labeling and risk management operate in silos, both are incomplete.

Closing the loop:

- Labeling engineers should participate in usability testing and contribute findings as foreseeable misuse inputs to the risk management file.
- Risk management should share hazard analyses early enough that high-severity hazards shape the IFU's information hierarchy — ensuring catastrophic-severity warnings receive appropriate prominence.

Labeling Complaints as Post-Market Safety Signals

Labeling complaints — user confusion, misinterpretation of warnings, failure to notice contraindications, difficulty following critical instructions — are **post-market safety inputs** with direct implications for the risk management file.

ISO 14971 Clause 10 requires systematic review of production and post-production information for implications to hazard identification, probability estimates, severity characterization, and risk control effectiveness.

For example: A complaint describing a user performing a step that a critical warning was supposed to have addressed, is evidence that the warning's **real-world effectiveness** does not match the effectiveness assumed during pre-market evaluation.

This is not merely a labeling quality issue. It is a **risk assessment signal**.

User Training as Verified Risk Control

When information for safety is implemented through **training** rather than written labeling, it becomes the most verifiable form of information for safety.

Training allows the manufacturer to observe user performance, confirm comprehension, identify misunderstandings, and verify competency before the device reaches a patient.

Under IEC 62366, training is recognized as a third-priority risk control option alongside information for safety — but with **higher verification expectations**.

The hazard analysis identifies **critical tasks** (tasks whose incorrect performance contributes to serious or catastrophic hazards) that can be candidates for rigorous training to demonstrate direct verification of competency.

For example: Biomedical engineers performing installation, servicing, or maintenance tasks — torque settings, electrical safety checks, flow verification — may be executing the final validation of a safety-critical function before patient use. Their training must be **commensurate with the severity of harm** if these tasks are performed incorrectly.

Training materials — procedure manuals, quick installation sheets, online modules, simulations — are design documents communicating safety messages. Like the IFU, they must:

- be evaluated against the risk management file,
- be verified for effectiveness when identified as risk controls,
- and be monitored during post-market surveillance.

An organization that designs training based on device complexity or commercial interest — rather than the **severity of patient harm** associated with each task — has built a training program that serves commercial goals, not patient safety obligations.

What Risk Management Actually Needs from You

Risk management needs labeling engineers, technical writers, and training developers to:

- **Recognize the IFU as a risk control measure.** Every warning, caution, contraindication, and limitation must trace to a documented residual risk.
- **Apply the distinction between information for safety and residual risk disclosure.** Only information for safety reduces risk; residual risk disclosure communicates transparency.
- **Ensure categorization is commensurate with severity.** High-severity hazards require warnings with appropriate prominence and placement.
- **Provide foreseeable misuse insights to the hazard analysis.** Usability findings and labeling-related complaints must flow into risk management.
- **Design training programs aligned with the hazard analysis.** Tasks with the highest severity consequences require the most rigorous training and competency verification.

- **Monitor labeling and training effectiveness post-market.** Complaints, user errors, and field feedback must be evaluated for implications to the risk management file.

Labeling and training are the final implementation of many risk controls. They are where the device's safety architecture meets the user — and ultimately, the patient.

Notes & Sources

- **On the specific IFU content categories and their relationship to residual risk** — ISO 20417:2021.
- **On the IFU and labeling as part of the user interface subject to usability engineering requirements** — IEC 62366-1:2015/AMD1:2020.
- **On FDA labeling requirements and the obligation to communicate safety information** — FDA, "Applying Human Factors and Usability Engineering to Medical Devices," 2016; 21 CFR Part 801.

Part V— Post-Market Functions

Chapter 25: Post-Market Surveillance

What This Part Is About

Part V of this book addresses the post-market phase — not as the end of the risk story, but as the place where the risk story is **continuously rewritten**. Every device on the market is generating evidence. Every patient who uses it, every clinician who reports a problem, every service technician who opens it, every publication that studies it, and every regulatory authority that issues a safety communication is providing data about whether the manufacturer's **pre-market risk assumptions were correct**.

That data does not automatically find its way into the risk management file. It must be intentionally and procedurally collected, assessed, and connected to specific hazardous situations and risk control assumptions. The organizational system that performs this work is **post-market surveillance (PMS)**. The function that often owns it is Post-Market Quality (PMQ), though in practice the data feeding it comes from nearly every function in the organization.

This chapter introduces the PMS system as a whole: what it is, what it is supposed to do, where its data comes from, and what its outputs mean for the risk management file. The chapters that follow — complaints handling, service and field support, and corrections and recalls — address the specific functions that feed this system. This chapter provides the framework within which each of those functions makes sense.

The Risk Management File Is Not Finished at Launch

The risk management file contains the manufacturer's best pre-market assessment of hazards, risks, risk controls, and the benefit–risk balance. At the time of market release, it reflected everything the manufacturer knew. It does **not** reflect what the manufacturer will learn.

Real patients in real clinical environments are not the same as subjects in controlled pre-market studies. Clinical populations are more diverse, more complex, and more vulnerable. Use environments are noisier, more demanding, and less controlled. Clinicians use devices in ways that are foreseeable but not anticipated. Patients use devices in ways that are understandable but not predicted.

Examples include:

- Emerging literature that changes the accepted understanding of a hazard category.
- A supplier change that subtly shifts a safety-critical characteristic.
- A competing device experiencing a failure mode that reveals a hazard all equivalent manufacturers must characterize.

All of this information is relevant to whether the device's risk conclusions — probability estimates, severity characterizations, and residual risk determinations — remain valid.

ISO 14971:2019 Clause 10 requires manufacturers to establish a system to **actively** collect and review this information. "Actively" is deliberate: the manufacturer cannot wait for information to arrive. A PMS program that only processes incoming complaints is reactive. ISO 14971 requires something more — a **proactive, systematic, ongoing** process of seeking out information that could affect the accuracy of the risk management file.

Clause 10 requires manufacturers to be able to answer four questions at any time:

1. Have any previously unrecognized hazards been identified from post-market experience?
2. Has the estimated risk from any characterized hazardous situation changed such that it is no longer within acceptable levels?
3. Has the overall residual risk become unacceptable in light of new evidence?

4. Has the original risk assessment been invalidated by new information? For example, changes in the state of the art may alter what constitutes acceptable practice for managing a particular hazard.

These four questions define the governing purpose of the PMS system. Every data source, every trend, every signal ultimately exists to help answer these questions for every device on the market. And every time one of these questions yields an affirmative answer, the risk management file must be updated and re-evaluated — and the manufacturer must determine whether any action is required.

Why this matters: A risk management file that is not continuously updated becomes a historical document, not a safety document. PMS is the mechanism that keeps it alive.

What Feeds the PMS System

Most practitioners, when asked what data sources PMS includes, begin with complaints. Complaints are important — and the subject of Chapter 26 — but they are only one input among many. A PMS system designed primarily around complaints will miss the signals that appear first in other channels.

A mature PMS system incorporates a broad range of data sources:

Complaints and adverse event reports: Direct communications from clinicians, patients, distributors, and healthcare facilities describing problems with the device. These are the most visible and most frequently cited in regulatory frameworks.

Service and repair records: Findings from field service visits, preventive maintenance, and repairs. For example, a technician replacing a component that has worn in an unexpected pattern; a device operating outside its calibrated range; a repair performed earlier than expected in the device's service life.

These are PMS signals — yet most organizations do not systematically connect service records to PMS or the risk management file.

Production nonconformances and process trend data: In-process inspection results, outgoing inspection trends, and production deviation patterns can reveal whether a risk control is being reliably implemented. For example, a rising trend in nonconformances for a safety-critical characteristic may indicate that the probability assumptions in the risk file are drifting.

CAPA outcomes and recurrence data: Whether corrective actions have been effective — and whether problems addressed by prior CAPAs are recurring — is post-market evidence about whether root causes of safety-relevant problems have truly been resolved.

Scientific and clinical literature: New publications can:

- reveal previously unrecognized hazards,
- provide incidence rate data that changes probability estimates,
- describe failure modes not previously characterized,
- or shift the state of the art in ways that change what constitutes acceptable risk.

ISO 14971 requires that the state of the art be considered — and the state of the art evolves continuously.

Clinical registries and real-world evidence: Where registries exist, they provide long-term outcomes data at a scale and duration pre-market studies cannot match. For example, implant revision rates over 10 years, complication rates across thousands of patients, real-world performance in subpopulations underrepresented in trials, and so on.

Regulatory authority communications: Safety alerts, field safety notices, guidance documents, and database communications from FDA, EU competent authorities,

MHRA, Health Canada, TGA, and others. For example, a safety alert about a competitor device using the same technology, or MAUDE trends for comparable devices, EUDAMED summaries (when it becomes fully operational), and so on.

Supplier quality signals: Incoming inspection trends, supplier nonconformance rates, and supplier change notifications. A supplier whose process has drifted is creating a patient safety signal that should reach PMS **before** it becomes a complaint.

Cybersecurity vulnerability disclosures: For connected devices, newly disclosed vulnerabilities in software components listed in the device's SBOM are post-market information. If a vulnerability affects a safety-critical function, probability estimates must be reassessed.

User feedback from technical support, training, and sales: Examples include use error patterns observed during training, labeling confusion reported to technical support, field observations from clinical sales representatives, etc.

These informal channels are often the **earliest indicators** of emerging safety issues.

Post-market clinical follow-up (PMCF) outputs: PMCF activities under EU MDR generate structured clinical evidence that feeds into the CER and PSUR. This evidence must be evaluated for its implications to the risk management file.

Why this matters: A PMS system built only around complaints sees only the problems that have already reached patients. A PMS system built around all available data sources sees the problems **before** they reach patients.

The Risk-Based Decisions in PMS

The PMQ professional who owns the PMS system is not primarily a data collector. They are a **decision-maker**. The data collection infrastructure exists to support a series of risk-based decisions that determine whether the device's risk conclusions remain valid and whether patients remain adequately protected.

1. Signal detection: Is this a data point or a signal?

Not every complaint, literature finding, or service report indicates a shift in the risk profile. Escalation thresholds must be **commensurate with risk.**

For example:

- A single complaint involving a catastrophic failure mode requires immediate action.
- A single complaint about packaging aesthetics does not.

2. Trend determination: Is this signal becoming a pattern?

Trending requires a benchmark — which is the occurrence rate estimated in the risk management file.

The question is: **Does the observed frequency match the probability predicted in the current risk assessment?** Trending without a benchmark identifies patterns. Trending **with** a benchmark identifies a shift in patient safety and device risk profile.

Why this matters: These decisions are where PMS stops being a reporting function and becomes a **patient safety function.**

The PMS System and the Risk Management File: The Loop That Must Close

The essential test of a PMS system is not whether it collects data. It is whether the data it collects:

- reaches the risk management file,
- triggers risk re-evaluations when appropriate,
- and leads to action when needed.

A PMS system that generates reports, identifies trends, escalates signals, and concludes analyses **without explicitly evaluating against the risk management file** is producing documentation — not closing the loop.

The traceability — from PMS finding → risk evaluation → escalation or action — is the evidentiary record that demonstrates that risk management is genuinely ongoing rather than a pre-market exercise.

The chapters that follow address the specific organizational functions that feed the PMS system with their most important data. All of them feed the same system. All of them serve the same purpose: **keeping the risk assessments honest with what is happening to patients and users in the field.**

Notes & Sources

- **On the obligation to actively collect and review production and post-production information** — ISO 14971:2019, Clause 10.
- **On the technical guidance for implementing a PMS system consistent with ISO 13485 and ISO 14971** — ISO/TR 20416:2020.
- **On the EU MDR structured PMS obligations** — EU MDR 2017/745, Articles 83–86; Annex III.
- **On FDA post-market surveillance requirements** — 21 CFR Part 822.

Chapter 26: Complaints Handling & Complaints Intake

Low complaint volume feels like good news. But low complaint volume and genuine product safety are not the same thing. A manufacturer with few complaints may indeed be producing a device that works reliably and rarely harms patients. Or they may be producing a device with real safety issues — but their complaints process is failing to detect them.

This distinction is critical to the risk management file. A risk management file updated with complete, accurately coded complaint data and reliable patient-impact information reflects the device's **actual** safety performance. A risk management file updated with missed reports, vague codes, and incomplete patient involvement information reflects the organization's **ability to capture complaints**, not the device's safety profile.

These are not the same thing. A manufacturer who cannot tell them apart is managing the **appearance** of safety, not safety itself.

This chapter is about the specific decisions that complaint handlers and intake specialists make every day — decisions that determine which of those two realities their organization inhabits, and what those decisions mean for product risk and ultimately patient safety.

What Complaint Handlers and Intake Specialists Actually Do

The complaint function spans several interconnected roles:

- **Intake specialists** receive initial reports from customers, clinicians, patients, distributors, and sales representatives.
- **Complaint investigators** examine events in depth — reviewing returned devices, interviewing reporters, analyzing manufacturing records, and determining root causes.

- **Trending analysts** aggregate complaint records over time, looking for patterns that individual complaints cannot reveal.
- **Post-market quality engineers** oversee the system as a whole, ensuring that its outputs reach the PMS program and, through it, the risk management file.

What all of these roles share is this: **they are the front door of the post-market evidence base.**

Why this matters: If the front door is narrow, misaligned, or poorly constructed, the entire post-market safety system receives distorted information — and the risk management file becomes fiction rather than evidence.

Section One: The Intake Decision

Every Customer-Facing Employee Is an Intake Point

The complaint clock — the regulatory timeline governing how quickly a complaint must be evaluated, investigated, and potentially reported — starts **not** when a record is created in the complaint database, but when the manufacturer becomes aware of the issue.

FDA and ISO 13485 are explicit on this point.

A clinical sales specialist who hears from a surgeon that a device stopped working during a procedure… A technical support representative who receives a call describing unexpected device behavior… A field service technician told by a biomedical engineer that the same device failed twice in a month…

Each of these individuals is the manufacturer's **point of awareness**. The countdown begins at the moment of that conversation — not when the complaint record is eventually created.

A surgeon describing a malfunction during surgery is making a complaint — even if they never use the word "complaint." A biomedical engineer calling about a failure during installation testing is also making a complaint.

The risk-based decision at this moment is not whether the reporter framed their message as a complaint. It is whether the message points to a **potential flaw in the device**.

Was There Patient Involvement?

The most crucial aspect of an intake interview is determining whether a patient was involved — and if so, what happened to them. Patient involvement is the **first severity signal**.

Two identical device failures can have radically different risk implications:

- A device that malfunctions **inside a patient's body** during a procedure
- The same device malfunctioning **during bench testing** in a biomedical engineering lab

The failure mode is identical. The risk is not.

The intake interview must therefore capture:

- Was the device being used on a patient at the time?
- Did any harm occur?
- What type of harm?
- Was clinical intervention required?
- Did the patient experience delayed harm or follow-up complications?

Why this matters: If patient involvement is missed or poorly documented, every downstream decision — investigation depth, MDR determination, trending thresholds — becomes mis-calibrated.

What Exactly Failed, and How?

The complaint code assigned during intake determines whether the failure mode can be trended against the risk analysis. A complaint coded as **"Device malfunction – General"** will never trend against the specific hazardous situation it represents.

A complaint coded as:

- "Pump occlusion – distal line – during infusion"
- "Battery failure – premature depletion – during transport"
- "Sensor drift – temperature probe – after sterilization cycle"

…can be trended against the correct hazard in the risk management file.

For example: A pump occlusion coded as "General malfunction" disappears into noise. A pump occlusion coded as "Occlusion – distal line – during infusion" becomes visible in trend analysis — and can trigger a risk-based escalation.

Why this matters: Mis-coding hides safety-critical failure modes. Accurate coding is the bridge between complaints and risk management.

Section Two: From Record to Risk Management File

What Investigation Must Answer

A complaint investigation is a characterization of:

- what actually happened,
- why it happened,
- and what it means for the device's safety profile.

A complete investigation must establish the failure mode with enough specificity to connect the event to a **characterized hazardous situation** in the risk management file. Examples of questions investigators must answer:

- Did the device fail to deliver its intended therapeutic output?
- Did the device behave in a way **outside** the failure modes considered in the risk file?
- Did the clinical context amplify harm in ways the hazard analysis did not anticipate?
- Did the sequence of events unfold more rapidly than predicted?

The risk-based question is: **Given this root cause and this failure mode, what does the risk management file say — and does it still apply?**

If what happened was worse than predicted — i.e., higher severity, faster progression, more vulnerable patient population — the risk must be re-assessed. If a failure mode materialized that the risk file never characterized, the hazard analysis must be expanded.

Both outcomes require investigations specific enough to make that comparison.

MDR Reportability as a Risk Management Assessment

The Medical Device Reporting (MDR) determination under 21 CFR 803 is one of the most consequential risk-based decisions. The MDR standard asks: **If this malfunction recurred, would it likely cause or contribute to serious injury or death?**

This cannot be answered without referencing the risk management file. A malfunction that caused **no harm in this event** may still be MDR-reportable if the risk file characterizes the potential consequences as serious.

For example: A defibrillator battery fails during testing in the hospital's biomedical lab. No patient was involved. No harm occurred.

But the risk file states that battery failure during emergency use could lead to death. And that's why this event is MDR-reportable.

An MDR investigator who evaluates only the complaint narrative — without linking the failure mode to the hazardous situation and severity in the risk file — is not completing a full evaluation.

Why this matters: Failing to identify a reportable adverse event is not only a regulatory violation — it is a failure to alert leadership to a safety concern identified in their own data.

Section Three: Trending as Risk Management Infrastructure

The Denominator Problem

A complaint is an event. A trend is a **rate**. The difference is the denominator: the number of devices in the field, in the relevant time period, for the device type being tracked.

Three complaints in a fleet of 5,000 devices is not the same as three complaints in a fleet of 50. Trending without denominators compares complaint counts to each other — revealing only whether volume is rising or falling. It does not reveal whether real-world performance is consistent with predicted occurrence rates.

Denominator data — typically owned by manufacturing, regulatory, or marketing — must be systematically available to appropriately assess risk.

Risk-Based Thresholds

Trending thresholds that trigger escalation must be commensurate with risk. For example:

- A failure mode associated with a **catastrophic** hazardous situation should have a **very low** threshold.
- A failure mode associated with **minor, reversible harm** can tolerate a higher threshold.

Setting the same threshold for both — often because the trending procedure was written without reference to severity — treats safety-critical failure modes with the same urgency as cosmetic ones.

This complies with the requirement to trend, while failing the obligation to protect patients. The trending function and risk management team must collaborate to:

- map each complaint code to its corresponding hazardous situation,
- identify the severity characterization,
- and set thresholds accordingly.

This link is what makes trend analysis a **true risk-based process**.

When Trending Triggers a Risk Management File Update

The output of trending is not a report on complaint volume. It is an assessment of whether the **probability estimates remain valid**. When trending reveals that the observed rate of a failure mode exceeds the pre-market probability estimate, the risk must be re-evaluated.

Explicit benefit–risk linkage: In some cases, complaint patterns may not only change probability estimates — they may challenge the **original benefit–risk conclusion**, especially for vulnerable patient subgroups.

For example:

- A device that performs well in adults but shows higher-than-expected complication rates in pediatric patients.
- A device whose benefit is lower than expected in a specific comorbidity group.

- A device whose real-world usability issues reduce its effective benefit in high-stress clinical environments.

Trending must escalate these findings with enough specificity to enable risk re-evaluation — and, when necessary, field action (which is discussed further in Chapter 28).

What Risk Management Actually Needs From You

Risk management needs the complaints process to understand that it is fundamentally about **evidence collection**. It needs:

- **Accurate intake.** Every message that points to a device flaw must be captured — regardless of whether the reporter uses the word "complaint."
- **Precise coding.** Failure modes must be coded specifically enough to trend against the risk file.
- **Patient involvement clarity.** Severity begins with understanding what happened to the patient.
- **Investigations tied to the risk file.** Root causes and failure modes must be compared to characterized hazardous situations.
- **MDR decisions grounded in risk.** Reportability depends on what *could* happen if the malfunction recurred — not just what happened this time.
- **Trending with denominators and risk-based thresholds.** Escalation criteria must be commensurate with severity.
- **Recognition that complaint patterns can challenge benefit–risk.** Especially for vulnerable subgroups.
- **A closed loop back to the risk management file.** Every validated trend must be evaluated for its implications to probability, severity, and benefit–risk.

Quality of complaint data determines the quality of safety decisions — whether residual risk is acceptable, whether field action is required, and most importantly, whether patient safety is protected.

Chapter 27: Service & Field Support

Part One: Service Personnel as Users

Who Gets Included in the Hazard Analysis

One of the most consequential decisions in any risk analysis is defining **who the users are.** In risk management, "users" are not limited to clinicians who operate the device during patient care. They include **every person who interacts with the device in ways that could expose them to harm or affect the device's safety performance.**

For devices designed to be maintained, calibrated, or repaired, this includes the people who:

- open the device,
- replace components,
- clean and disinfect assemblies,
- recalibrate instruments,
- and return the device to service.

IEC 62366-1, the usability engineering standard aligned with ISO 14971, requires manufacturers to identify **all user groups** as part of defining intended use. User groups differ in training, knowledge, environment, and interaction patterns — and therefore introduce different hazardous situations.

Clinical users — nurses, surgeons, physicians, patients — are always identified. Service users — OEM field service engineers, hospital biomedical equipment technicians, third-party repair technicians — often are not.

When service personnel are not defined as users, they are absent from the hazard analysis. Hazardous situations that arise **specifically during service activities** — electrical exposure from stored energy, biological contamination from prior patient use, bypassed interlocks during calibration — are simply not characterized.

EU MDR requires manufacturers to design equipment for safe servicing and to make relevant information accessible to authorized personnel. ISO 14971 Annex C identifies electrical, mechanical, radiological, and biological hazards — all of which may be encountered during maintenance — whether or not the manufacturer has assessed them.

Why this matters: If service personnel are not defined as users, the hazards they face — and the hazards they can create for patients — are invisible to the risk management file.

Hazardous Situations Related to Servicing Activities

Servicing introduces two categories of foreseeable hazardous situations, both equally important and often overlooked.

1. Hazards from the device to the service personnel

Examples include:

- An electrosurgical unit containing stored capacitive energy that can cause electrical shock if not properly discharged.
- An imaging instrument with radioactive components that may expose the technician if interlocks are disabled during calibration.
- A device with an accessible fluid path contaminated from prior patient use, creating a biological hazard.

Each scenario is a sequence of events in which the technician's interaction with the device exposes them to harm. The **severity and probability** of that harm must be characterized in the risk management file, and risk controls identified — inherent safe service design, protective measures, or information for safety in the form of clear service procedures.

2. Hazards created for subsequent patients

Service activities can also introduce hazards **for the next patient:**

- A mis-calibrated sensor

- A bypassed interlock
- A contaminated internal pathway
- A mis-installed component
- A configuration reset that undoes a clinical safety decision

Both categories belong in the hazard analysis because both represent real safety obligations.

Why this matters: If service-related hazards are not characterized, the organization is blind to risks that can arise **only** during maintenance — and blind to risks that maintenance can create.

The Service Manual as a Risk Control Measure

When service technicians are recognized as users, the service manual becomes more than a technical reference. It becomes a **risk control measure** — information for safety.

The service procedures are then required to be locatable, comprehensible, executable under real-world conditions, and clearly differentiated between safety-critical and non-critical steps.

Service work is often performed under time pressure, in clinical environments, without supervision, and with competing operational demands.

The usability of the service manual — whether warnings are prominent, whether restoration steps are unmistakable, whether safety-critical tasks are clearly marked — determines the **effectiveness of the risk controls** it implements.

Why this matters: A service manual that is unusable under real-world conditions is a failed risk control, no matter how complete it is on paper.

Part Two: Every Service Activity Is a Risk Control Interaction

What Preventive Maintenance Actually Is

Preventive maintenance (PM) is not merely upkeep. It is the periodic verification that **risk controls remain effective**. Risk controls designed into the device — dimensional tolerances, interlocks, filters, calibration parameters — drift over time. Components wear. Calibration shifts. Filters load with particulate.

The PM interval is the manufacturer's determination of how long these risk controls can remain effective before the **probability of failure approaches an unacceptable level**.

A correctly executed PM typically:

- replaces specified wear components,
- recalibrates parameters to within specified ranges,
- verifies safety-critical functions,
- and confirms the device's return to its specified condition.

The rigor of PM verification and the strictness of acceptance criteria must be **commensurate with the risk** associated with the functions being checked.

For example, a torque value on a pressure-sealing connector is not the same as a torque value on a housing screw.

Manufacturer responsibilities: Manufacturers must design PM procedures that:

- make safety-critical steps visible,
- specify non-negotiable acceptance criteria,
- and include post-service verification steps that confirm restoration of safety-critical functions.

Technician responsibilities: Once the distinction is visible, technicians must apply the additional care and precision that safety-critical steps require.

Why this matters: PM is the mechanism that keeps risk controls functioning. If PM is weak, inconsistent, or ambiguous, the risk management file becomes inaccurate — and patient safety erodes silently.

The Non-OEM Parts Problem

Every component in a medical device was selected, qualified, and characterized during design. Residual risk conclusions were based on **those specific components**. A non-OEM part substituted during repair changes the device in ways that were **never assessed.**

The risk-based question at every repair is: Does this replacement part preserve the residual risk conclusions established for the original component?

A field service engineer who substitutes a non-OEM part because the OEM part is back-ordered is making a **design change in the field**. Such substitutions must feed into change control and design control, because they alter the assumptions underlying the risk management file.

Why this matters: Residual risk conclusions apply only to the components evaluated. A non-OEM part invalidates those conclusions unless equivalence is established.

Software, Parameters, and Configuration

Modern devices contain configurable software — alarm thresholds, mode settings, workflow configurations. A service visit that resets parameters or deploys a software update is interacting with risk controls, often invisibly.

Alarm thresholds are a clear example. Factory defaults may be chosen for general populations. But hospitals may adjust thresholds for specific patient groups. Those adjustments are **clinical safety decisions.**

A service event that resets thresholds to factory defaults without restoring institution-specific settings has **undone a clinical safety decision**.

For example: Restoring factory alarm thresholds on a neonatal monitor after a software update may erase carefully chosen settings that protected premature infants from delayed detection of deterioration.

The service engineer may have no visibility into which parameters were configured or why. If service procedures do not require documenting and restoring configurations, the connection between technical service and clinical safety is lost.

Software patches must also be treated as design changes and subjected to risk analysis. A patch that fixes one issue but alters alarm behavior, dose calculation, or diagnostic accuracy may replace one hazardous situation with another.

Why this matters: Configuration resets and software updates can silently undo risk controls — unless service procedures explicitly prevent it.

The Urgency-Safety Tension

One of the most common hazards in service is not mechanical or technical — it is situational. A device is needed **now**.

The ICU patient needs the infusion pump. The OR team is waiting for the electrosurgical unit. The NICU nurse needs the ventilator.

The clinical consequences of device unavailability are immediate and real.

The decision to return a device to service **before full repair is complete** is a critical and often overlooked risk-based decision. The service engineer must understand which device capabilities are safety-critical and must refer to the risk management file to determine whether partial restoration is acceptable.

Why this matters: Urgency does not eliminate risk — it magnifies it. Decisions made under pressure must still be commensurate with risk of that feature.

Part Three: Service Records as Post-Market Evidence

Service Findings as the Earliest Signal

Service findings often appear **before** user complaints. A component approaching failure generates out-of-spec measurements, or increased wear, or early replacement at PM, or unusual calibration drift, long before it generates a patient-facing event.

Service records are **leading indicators**. Complaints are **lagging indicators**. Service records are part of the **ISO 14971 Clause 10 production and post-production information** that must be systematically collected and reviewed.

A mature organization asks:

- Are failure modes found during PM exceeding predicted probabilities?
- Are components wearing in ways not characterized in the hazard analysis?
- Are technicians encountering use conditions not captured in intended use?
- Are certain users experiencing more severe or more frequent failures?

In some cases, service findings may reveal that certain user subgroups experience more frequent or more severe failures — challenging the **original benefit–risk conclusion** for those populations.

Why this matters: If you wait for complaints, you learn about safety issues at the point of patient impact. Service findings let you learn **before** patients or users are harmed.

What Risk Management Actually Needs from You

Risk management needs field service engineers and biomedical equipment technicians to understand that their work is not independent of the risk management file — it is a **field-side interaction with it**.

Every PM step, every component replacement, every calibration adjustment, every software update either **maintains or alters** the context in which residual risks were assessed. Risk management needs:

- Service procedures that make safety-critical steps visible and mandatory
- PM rigor commensurate with severity
- Documentation and restoration of configuration settings
- Non-OEM substitutions treated as design changes
- Service findings escalated as post-production information to the risk file
- Early signals communicated before they become complaints

When service findings that affect safety are not conveyed back to update the risk management file, the organization's risk-based decisions drift away from actual product risk.

Service is not a technical function operating in isolation. It is a safety function — one that maintains, modifies, and reveals the real-world performance of the device.

Chapter 28: Corrections, Removals & Recall Management

This chapter is about the specific ways the corrections and removals function interacts with the product risk management file — what it takes from it, what it contributes to it, and what risk-based decisions it makes every day.

The corrections and removals team — sometimes called the field actions team, sometimes embedded in post-market quality or regulatory affairs — owns the process that begins when a potential safety signal escalates to the point where action on distributed devices may be required. The team evaluates whether that threshold has been crossed, determines what action is appropriate, defines the scope, communicates it, executes it, and verifies that it worked.

Every one of these activities is a **risk management activity**. Each requires the product risk management file as its primary analytical input. And each produces a risk-based conclusion — either that action was taken to restore acceptable residual risk, or that residual risk remained acceptable without action — that must be documented as such.

Section One: The Field Action Trigger Is a Risk Management Conclusion

What ISO 14971 Says About When Action Is Required

ISO 14971:2019 Clause 10 establishes the governance for when production and post-production information requires re-evaluating risk and taking further action. When the accumulation of PMS data, complaint trends, MDR investigations, service findings, or any other post-market evidence leads to:

- a previously unrecognized hazard,
- a probability estimate being exceeded,

- an overall residual risk becoming unacceptable, or
- the original assessment being otherwise invalidated,

the manufacturer is obligated to respond. The nature and urgency of that response must be **commensurate with the severity and probability** of the affected hazardous situation.

This is the direct linkage between ISO 14971 and corrections and removals. Clause 10 is the decision framework. A corrections and removals team that begins its evaluation by asking, "What does the risk management file say about this hazardous situation, and does the evidence we have change that picture?" is applying the framework correctly. A team that begins by asking, "Is this a Class I or a Class II?" has skipped the analysis and gone straight to regulatory classification — which is a **downstream output** of the risk assessment, not a substitute for it.

Why this matters: If the trigger is treated as a classification exercise instead of a risk assessment, the organization can comply on paper while failing patients in practice.

The Health Hazard Evaluation Is an ISO 14971 Analysis

The formal mechanism for evaluating whether a field action is required — and if so, what kind — is the Health Hazard Evaluation (HHE). Under FDA's recall framework, the HHE assesses:

- severity of the health hazard,
- probability of occurrence,
- patient populations at risk,
- and whether injuries have already occurred.

Under EU MDR, the Field Safety Corrective Action (FSCA) framework requires assessment of whether the risk of the field action itself outweighs the risk of leaving the device in use.

These assessments use the same analytical dimensions as ISO 14971: severity, probability, population characteristics, and benefit–risk trade-offs. The product risk management file is the primary input because that work has already been done. The hazard analysis has characterized failure modes and hazardous situations, the severity of potential harm, and the probability of occurrence based on pre-market evidence.

The HHE does not reconstruct this from scratch. It asks:

- Has the observed event rate exceeded the pre-market probability estimate?
- Has a clinical consequence occurred that is more severe than characterized?
- Has a risk control been found non-functional in the field in ways the residual risk analysis did not anticipate?

When the HHE's severity or probability assessments differ from the risk management file, that difference must be explained and documented. Either:

- the original risk assessment was incorrect and must be updated,
- the post-market evidence reveals a new pattern, or
- the field event and the characterized hazardous situation differ in ways that legitimately affect the assessment.

In all cases, the risk management file must be updated as part of the field action process — not afterward as a retrospective documentation exercise, but as an integral part of the decision-making itself.

Why this matters: Effectively, the HHE is an ISO 14971 analysis performed in the post-market context. If it is disconnected from the risk management file, the organization is making high-stakes decisions without its own best evidence.

The Decision Not to Act Is Also a Risk-Based Decision

One of the most consequential and most overlooked realities is that the decision **not** to initiate a field action — the conclusion that post-market evidence does not require action — is itself a **risk acceptance decision**. It is a documented conclusion that:

- the residual risk characterizations in the risk management file remain valid, and
- continued patient exposure to the device in its current form is within acceptable risk levels.

This conclusion must be documented with the same rigor as a decision to act. 21 CFR Part 806 requires records for corrections and removals that are not required to be reported, including the justification for why no report was required. The level of analysis and documentation supporting a "no action" decision must be **commensurate with the safety risk** associated with the failure mode.

Organizations that resolve borderline issues through informal discussions — "this isn't serious enough to warrant a field action" — without a written risk assessment explaining how that determination was reached, are making risk acceptance decisions without evidence that patient safety considerations drove the result.

What matters in this record is patient safety responsibility. If the same failure later leads to an adverse event, the critical questions will be: What was known? When was it known? How was the risk assessment justified in determining no action was necessary? There must be a written record that reflects the nature of the risk and shows how patient safety considerations drove the determination.

Why this matters: The most dangerous decision is often the one that leaves the device unchanged while the risk has changed.

Section Two: Three Field Action Decisions That Are Risk Acceptance Decisions

Once the decision to initiate a field action has been made, the corrections and removals team faces three consequential choices. All three are risk-based decisions. All three require the product risk management file as a primary input.

Decision One: What Type of Action?

The nature of the field action — be it a software patch, label change, advisory, retrieval, replacement, or a combination — dictates the type of risk control the company is applying in response to the identified risk.

This selection must follow the same order of precedence outlined in ISO 14971 for any risk control decision:

1. Inherent safety by design
2. Protective measures
3. Information for safety

The rigor and intrusiveness of the field action must be **commensurate with the severity and probability** of the hazardous situation.

When a design-level correction is not yet feasible, an interim communication — a field safety notice, use advisory, or temporary instruction — may be appropriate as a **bridge**. It is an information-for-safety response: it reduces the probability of harm by modifying user behavior rather than changing the device. This is the lowest tier of the risk control hierarchy and is appropriate:

- as a temporary measure while a design correction is developed, or
- for failure modes where the hazardous situation is primarily use-related and information genuinely changes the risk picture.

It is **not** appropriate as the primary and permanent response to a high-severity failure mode rooted in device design.

Example: A design flaw in a life-sustaining device that can cause sudden loss of function cannot be addressed solely with a use advisory. The risk management file's severity characterization demands a design correction and device replacement, not just information for safety.

There is an additional dimension under EU MDR FSCA: the obligation to weigh the risk of the field action itself against the risk of continued use. For a device managing a life-threatening condition, physically removing it from clinical use to perform a correction may expose patients to greater immediate harm than the defect being corrected. In such cases, the **benefit–risk characterization** is directly relevant. The field action decision is not only about reducing risk; it is about preserving an acceptable benefit–risk balance when removal of the device could itself harm patients.

Why this matters: If the type of action is chosen for regulatory convenience rather than commensurate with risk, the organization may appear responsive while leaving patients exposed.

Decision Two: What Is the Scope?

Scope determination — which units are included in the field action — directly determines how many patients are protected and how many remain at risk.

Scope too narrow leaves patients with affected devices unprotected. Whereas, scope too broad removes devices from patients who critically need them and may create new risks.

There are two aspects to scope:

1. **Technical scope:** The underlying failure mechanism must be understood well enough to determine which manufacturing periods, which software versions, which component lots, etc. can exhibit the failure mode.

   For example, failure modes associated with a specific software version affect only devices running that version; failures tied to certain component lots affect only devices containing those lots.

2. **Risk-oriented scope:** Here, severity is the calibration point. When severity is catastrophic, scope decisions must err on the side of conservatism proportional to that level of harm:

   - When it is unclear whether a borderline lot is affected, include it.
   - When traceability data is incomplete, expand scope to cover the uncertainty.

For low-severity failure modes, a tighter scope grounded in confirmed evidence may be appropriate.

For example: If a catastrophic failure mode may affect devices manufactured between January and March, but records are unclear for late March, a conservative, risk-commensurate decision is to include the borderline March units rather than exclude them.

The severity characterization in the risk management file for the affected hazardous situation tells the corrections and removals team which conservatism standard applies.

Why this matters: Scope is where conservatism — or lack of it — shows up as patient impact.

Decision Three: What Does the Communication Say?

The risk management file's characterization of the hazardous situation should directly govern the content of the communication. The communication must:

- describe the failure mode in terms clinical users can act on,
- explain under what conditions it occurs,
- articulate what it means for patient safety, and
- specify what the user must do – i.e., continue using the device with precautions, or stop using it immediately, or monitor previously treated patients, or take other defined actions.

A communication that explains the technological problem but not the clinical impact fails the information-for-safety obligation.

For example: A field safety notice that says, *"A firmware malfunction may impair battery charge calculations,"* informs the user about the technical issue. It does **not** tell them that:

- the device may suddenly stop working during use,
- this could delay therapy or monitoring,
- and this may result in serious harm or death.

The risk assessment — sudden malfunction, delayed response, potential adverse effects — is what gives the communication its clinical meaning.

Why this matters: If the communication does not translate the hazard into clinical terms and clear actions, it does not change behavior — and therefore does not change risk.

Section Three: The Risk Management File After the Field Action

Effectiveness Verification as Risk Control Verification

When the field action is complete — devices corrected, units retrieved, communications sent and acknowledged — the corrections and removals team is not finished. The field action implemented a **risk control**: a design correction, an advisory, a replacement.

Like any risk control, its effectiveness must be verified. Did the action actually reduce the residual risk for the scenario to acceptable levels? Effectiveness verification has two dimensions:

- **Operational effectiveness**
    - Were all affected units corrected or retrieved?
    - Were all affected customers notified and confirmed?
    - What is the reconciliation rate?
- **Clinical/safety effectiveness**
    - Did the software update eliminate the failure mode?
    - Did the replacement component restore performance to within acceptable limits?
    - Did the advisory change user behavior in the intended way?

Effectiveness verification for field actions is the **ISO 14971 requirement to verify that risk controls are implemented and effective**, applied in the post-market context.

This verification produces the output that closes the risk assessment loop: confirmation that residual risk for the affected hazardous situation has been restored to acceptable levels, and documented evidence that the risk control implemented through the field action is effective.

Why this matters: A field action that is not verified for effectiveness is a risk control in name only.

Updating the Risk Management File

A living risk management file throughout this process serves future decisions:

- If the same failure mode is observed again post-action, the file should show that it was previously characterized, addressed, and verified.
- If a similar failure mode appears in a product variant or subsequent generation, the record of the prior field action's analytical basis informs the new assessment.
- If a regulatory authority inspects the manufacturer's handling of the field action, the risk management file demonstrates the patient safety reasoning behind each decision.

Organizations that treat the risk management file as a pre-market document — complete at market release, archived until the next submission — will have a file that accurately describes the device **before** it reached patients, and nothing more. Field action updates, effectiveness verifications, revised probability estimates, and new risk controls will not appear unless they are deliberately integrated into the post-market process.

What Risk Management Actually Needs from You

Risk management needs the corrections and removals function to understand that **every field action decision is a risk acceptance decision** — including the decision not to act — and that the product risk management file is the analytical foundation for those decisions.

It also needs the risk management file to be updated when the field action is complete:

- what was found,
- what risk control was implemented,
- what effectiveness verification confirmed,
- and what the revised residual risk conclusion is.

The loop does not close unless someone closes it. The corrections and removals function is uniquely positioned to ensure that this feedback is captured — so that future decisions are grounded in the full, honest history of how the device has behaved in the field and how the organization has responded in the interest of patient safety.

Notes & Sources

- **On corrections and removals reporting requirements** — 21 CFR Part 806.
- **On recall classification based on health hazard assessment** — 21 CFR Part 7; 21 CFR Part 806.
- **On field safety corrective actions under EU MDR** — EU MDR 2017/745, Articles 87–89.

Part VI – The Connected Organization

Chapter 29: Executive Leadership

In many medical device organizations, risk management is treated as something that happens in the quality department. Risk engineers build the files. Quality leaders review them. Regulatory affairs use them for submissions. Risk management becomes a quality system process — governed by quality procedures, audited by quality auditors, and summarized at management review by the quality function.

Executive leadership — the CEO, the head of R&D, the VP of Operations, the commercial leader — may see a summary at management review or sign the risk management report before launch or submission. But outside those moments, the prevailing belief is that risk management "belongs to quality," and leadership's role is simply to empower quality to execute it.

In reality, **every risk-based decision described in this book operates inside a framework only executive leadership can define**. The risk policy that sets risk acceptance criteria is established by leadership. The residual risk conclusions that determine whether a device is acceptable for patient use are approved by leadership. The competence and resourcing of the people performing risk assessments are determined by leadership.

If that framework is strong, patient safety becomes the governing principle across the organization. If it is weak, ambiguous, under-resourced, or culturally unsupported, every downstream decision — from design to complaints to field actions — is compromised.

This chapter is about what executive leadership actually owns in product risk management, what decisions only they can make, and what patient safety requires from them.

What Executive Leadership Actually Owns

ISO 14971:2019 Section 4.2 places responsibility for establishing the risk policy explicitly with **top management**. This is not a delegated quality task. It is a named management obligation: top management shall define and document criteria for risk acceptability.

Section 4.3 assigns leadership responsibility for ensuring the competence of risk management personnel. The risk management report — the document that concludes overall residual risk acceptability before release — requires management approval. That signature is the moment leadership formally accepts, on behalf of the organization, that the residual risks remaining after all controls are applied are acceptable in light of the device's clinical benefits.

ISO 13485:2016 Clause 5 devotes an entire section to management responsibility. EU MDR Article 10(9) names management responsibility as a required element of the QMS. FDA's 2024 QMSR preamble states explicitly that executives must embrace a culture of quality as foundational to safe device manufacturing.

Across every framework — ISO 14971, ISO 13485, FDA, EU MDR — the message is consistent: **accountability for the adequacy of the risk management system cannot be delegated**. Functional teams execute risk management. Leadership is responsible for whether the system is adequate for the task.

Section One: The Risk Policy — The Constitutional Document of Patient Safety

What the Risk Policy Actually Is

The risk policy is the organization's documented statement of how it defines acceptable patient safety risk. It specifies:

- the severity and probability scales used in risk assessments,
- the risk acceptance criteria that determine which risks require control and how far,
- the threshold above which benefit–risk analysis is required,

- and the principles that ensure consistent application across the portfolio.

This document is created **before** any specific device is analyzed. It is leadership's commitment — in writing — to the standard of patient safety that will govern every product decision.

Once written, the risk policy constrains every future decision; it is the closest thing the organization has to a constitution for patient safety.

Why this matters: If the risk policy is weak, vague, or tailored to justify existing products, it cannot govern future decisions. It becomes a loophole, not a standard.

What the Risk Policy Must Specify — and Why It Is a Leadership Decision

Leadership must answer foundational questions:

- **What severity of harm is categorically unacceptable**, regardless of probability? (For most organizations, catastrophic harm — potential patient death — belongs here.)
- **What probability thresholds define tolerable vs. intolerable risk?** A manufacturer of high-risk implantable devices should have stricter thresholds than a manufacturer of low-risk diagnostics.
- **How is benefit–risk analysis conducted when residual risk remains above acceptable levels?** Leadership must define:
    - what constitutes clinical benefit,
    - how benefit is measured relative to residual risk,
    - who has authority to make benefit–risk decisions,
    - and what evidence is required.

These criteria must be defined **in advance**, not tailored to rescue a struggling product.

Why this matters: A risk policy written reactively — to justify a device already under pressure — defeats its purpose. It must be written with clarity, courage, and independence from commercial timelines.

Product Class, Patient Population, and the Calibration of Risk Criteria

Risk criteria must be calibrated to the portfolio:

- A manufacturer of Class I exam gloves and a manufacturer of Class III implantable cardiac devices cannot share the same risk acceptance criteria.
- Devices used in vulnerable populations — children, seniors, immunocompromised patients — require stricter criteria.
- Devices used in high-acuity environments require different thresholds than devices used occasionally in healthy adults.

The risk policy is therefore a **cross-functional leadership document**. Its calibration requires input from R&D, clinical, regulatory, quality, operations, and commercial leadership.

Section Two: Four Obligations That Only Leadership Can Fulfill

Obligation One: Resource the Risk Management Function Adequately

The most common form of executive failure in risk management is a **resource failure**. FDA warning letters consistently cite inadequate resources — insufficient personnel, inadequate competence, or quality functions without authority — as root causes of system breakdowns.

ISO 14971 requires leadership to ensure adequate resources and competence for risk management activities. Adequate resourcing means:

- enough competent people,
- with enough time,
- and enough authority,
- to perform rigorous risk assessments across the portfolio.

Resourcing of risk management must be **commensurate with the complexity and risk profile** of the portfolio.

Why this matters: Under-resourced risk management produces under-analyzed risk — and patients pay the price.

Obligation Two: Hold All Functional Leaders Accountable for Patient Safety Culture

ISO 14971 refers to "top management" generically, which often leads organizations to assume that risk management obligations belong to quality and regulatory alone. But the failures described throughout this book are cross-functional.

Leadership must communicate — clearly, consistently, and visibly — that patient safety is **every function's responsibility**. This is demonstrated not by policy statements but by leadership behavior:

- the questions asked at project reviews,
- the concerns escalated,
- the behaviors rewarded,
- and the shortcuts refused.

Why this matters: Culture is not created by procedures. It is created by what leaders pay attention to.

Obligation Three: Approve Residual Risk and Benefit-Risk Conclusions With Genuine Understanding

Management approval of the risk management report should not be a procedural signature. It should be an informed decision:

- What residual risks remain?
- What are the clinical consequences if they materialize?
- Why are these risks acceptable in light of the device's benefits?
- Is the evidence supporting the benefit–risk conclusion adequate?
- Do the conclusions fall within the risk policy?

The depth of leadership review must be **commensurate with the severity and irreversibility** of the harms being accepted. Benefit–risk decisions above certain thresholds should require explicit leadership review.

Obligation Four: Use Management Review as a Patient Safety Governance Mechanism

Management review is required by ISO 13485 and FDA QMSR. But in many organizations, it becomes a reporting exercise: quality presents data, leadership listens, minutes are taken. However, a management review that governs patient safety asks different questions:

- Not just how many complaints were received — but whether trending identified new failure modes not in the risk file.
- Not just how many CAPAs are open — but whether any involve safety-critical risk controls.

- Not just whether the PMS plan was executed — but whether PMS data revealed risks exceeding acceptable levels.
- Not just whether risk reports were approved — but whether residual risk conclusions remain valid given new evidence.

If management review does not change any decisions, priorities, or resource allocations, **it is reporting, not governance**.

Why this matters: Management review is the only recurring forum where leadership sees the full safety picture. If it is passive, the organization is not well-informed.

Section Three: The Tone That Flows Downstream

Every function described in this book contributes to the risk management file. What makes those contributions reliable is not the procedures they follow — it is the **culture they work within**.

Organizational culture is shaped by what leaders fund, what they ask about, what they escalate, what they reward, and what they refuse to accept.

When the head of R&D asks whether a change control evaluation was assessed for product risk, teams understand that patient safety is the priority. When a complaint trend suggests a field action may be needed, leadership must support investigation even when commercial timing is unfavorable. These are leadership behaviors. They are the living expression of the risk policy.

When top management promotes a strong safety culture, every function performs its daily responsibilities with a patient-safety-first mindset.

Our patients trust the system. They assume that the device placed in their body, used in their procedure, or monitoring their vital signs was manufactured by an organization that took their safety seriously at every level. That trust is honored — or broken — primarily by leadership decisions.

Chapter 30: Where the Handoffs Break Down

The Pattern That Runs Through Every Chapter

If you have read this book from the beginning, you have now encountered more than twenty functions in a medical device organization. You have seen the quality engineer, the systems engineer, the software developer, the human factors specialist, the biocompatibility engineer, the reliability engineer, the packaging engineer, the sterilization engineer, the regulatory affairs professional, the clinical scientist, the complaint handler, the service technician, the recall manager, and the executive. You have seen how each interacts with the product risk management file — what they contribute to it, what they take from it, and what risk-based decisions they make every day.

And you may have noticed something else: **similar failures appear in different forms in nearly every chapter.**

These are not failures of individual competence. In each case, the person involved was performing their own duties impeccably. The failure was systemic: knowledge held by one function did not reach another function that needed it, at the moment it mattered, in a form that could drive action.

This is the handoff problem. It is the most pervasive challenge in the medical device industry, and it almost never appears explicitly in warning letters or inspection findings. Regulators cite inadequate CAPA, deficient design controls, or weak post-market surveillance. But beneath each surface failure is a deeper one: **information that existed somewhere in the organization did not reach the right function to make a safe decision.**

This chapter names the most common handoff failures — drawn from the specific functions and moments described throughout this book — and offers a framework for understanding why they occur and what organizations can do to prevent them.

Part One: The Handoffs That Break Most Often

From Design to Manufacturing: The Transfer That Loses the Safety Rationale

Chapter 17 described design transfer. Many specifications established during design are **risk controls**: dimensional tolerances, material specifications, surface finishes, bonding procedures. These exist because the risk management file characterizes deviation from them as causes of hazardous situations.

The handoff breaks when manufacturing receives the specification **without the safety rationale**. They receive *what* is required, but not *why*. Without context, the manufacturing engineer applies equal flexibility to all specifications. A critical-to-safety dimension is treated the same as a cosmetic one.

Why this matters: When manufacturing does not know which specifications are safety-critical risk controls, patient safety becomes dependent on luck rather than design.

What the handoff requires: Design transfer must identify which specifications correspond to risk controls, with explicit reference to the hazardous situation. This is not a large addition — a column, a flag, a category — but it transforms a specification from a number on a drawing into a **patient safety threshold**.

From Clinical Evidence to the Hazard Analysis: The Severity Gap

Chapter 22 described clinical contribution to the risk analysis. Severity cannot be reliably assessed without clinical input. Questions such as:

- What is the expected outcome for a 70-year-old patient with comorbidities?

- How quickly does deterioration occur?
- What is the realistic clinical response time?

These are clinical questions, not engineering ones.

The handoff breaks when the hazard analysis does not include real-world clinical input. The engineer assesses severity using a generic idea of clinical impact — technically correct in an ideal scenario, but disconnected from the actual patient population and clinical environment.

Why this matters: Severity characterizations that are not grounded in clinical reality lead to risk controls that are not commensurate with the harm they are meant to prevent.

What the handoff requires: Medical affairs and clinical safety must be **formally integrated** into the risk management process — not as ad hoc reviewers, but as active participants in hazards identification and severity assessments.

From Post-Market Data to the Risk Management File: The Loop That Never Closes

This handoff failure appears throughout the book. For example:

- A service engineer finds a parameter out of specification during PM and documents it — but there is no procedure to route service records for safety signal analysis.
- A trending analyst identifies a pattern that exceeds the pre-market probability estimate — but has no defined pathway back to the risk management file.
- PMCF outputs identify new complications — but are not reviewed against the hazard analysis.

Information that should be re-evaluated for safety risk reaches the organization through some channel — complaints, service records, trending reports, clinical studies — and then stops.

Why this matters: When post-market data does not update the risk management file, the organization's risk assessments drift further from reality with every passing month.

What the handoff requires: A defined, procedural connection between every post-market data source and risk management — a structured process in which complaint trending, service findings, MDR investigations, and PMCF outputs are reviewed for their impact on product risk and ultimately patient safety.

From Design Changes to Risk Assessment: The Pre-Decided Assessment

This is the handoff failure that is most overlooked. For example, a project manager walks into a meeting with a design change assessment already completed, already concluded as "not safety-significant," and already approved. The assessment is pre-decided, the timeline is locked, and organizational pressure is to move forward.

Why this matters: When change control decisions are made before appropriately assessing for risk, the organization is not managing risk — it is only managing schedule.

What the handoff requires: Change control procedures must require explicit identification of how the change corresponds to the risk management file — a mandatory, traceable step with documented rationale.

From Risk Management to Every Other Function: The Training Gap

The handoffs above involve information failing to reach the risk management file. But there is an equally important failure in the opposite direction: **the risk management framework failing to reach the functions that need it**. For example:

- The manufacturing engineer who does not know which specifications are risk controls cannot prioritize them in MRB decisions.
- The service technician who does not know which parameters are safety-critical cannot understand why certain PM steps require more rigor.
- The program manager who cannot interpret a risk management file cannot recognize when a change control assessment is inadequate.

This is not a process training problem. It is a **framework training** problem.

Why this matters: Handoffs break when functions apply equal flexibility to all tasks instead of applying rigor **commensurate with the risk** of the associated hazardous situation.

What the handoff requires: Function-specific training on the risk management framework — not ISO 14971 awareness, but targeted education showing each function:

- what they contribute to the risk management file,
- what they must take from it,
- and which of their daily decisions are risk-based decisions in disguise.

This book aims to be one such training resource.

Part Two: Why the Handoffs Break

Understanding what the handoff failures are is not enough. Organizations need to understand why they persist despite everyone's genuine intention to do good work.

Organizational Silos Are Not Accidental

Medical device organizations are structured by function because specialization is efficient. Engineers with engineers. Clinicians with clinicians. Quality with quality. Each function develops its own language, processes, timing, and performance measures.

But the risk management file is inherently **cross-functional**. It requires:

- clinicians to characterize severity,
- engineers to identify hazards and risk controls,
- manufacturing to evaluate process risks,
- regulatory affairs to provide context,
- post-market teams to maintain feedback loops.

No single function has all the expertise required.

Without formal procedures defining roles, responsibilities, escalation points, and information flow, cross-functional collaboration becomes dependent on personal relationships and goodwill — both of which are fragile and inconsistent.

Why this matters: A risk management system is not a chain of tasks — **it is a circulatory system**. When one artery is blocked, the entire system suffers.

The Risk Management File Is Invisible to Most Functions

A deeper structural problem is that the risk management file is not, in most organizations, a document that most functions can easily access, navigate, or use.

When a document is inaccessible to the people who need it, they stop using it. They make decisions based on their own judgment, their own experience, and whatever information is most immediately available to them — which is usually not the risk management file. The handoffs break not because people choose to ignore the risk management framework, but because of lack of awareness and training on how to use this framework in daily decisions impacting the product.

Why this matters: When the risk file is invisible, risk-based decisions become intuition-based decisions.

Part Three: The Cost of Broken Handoffs

Broken handoffs can lead to:

- delayed field actions,
- mis-calibrated risk assessments,
- inconsistent design decisions,
- increased regulatory exposure,
- and ultimately, preventable patient harm.

These are not theoretical consequences. They are the root causes of many of the industry's most serious failures.

Part Four: What Organizations Can Do

Make the Risk Management File Navigable

The risk management file must be easily searchable and usable by the functions that depend on it. Modern QMS, digital transformation tools and integrated risk systems make this possible. For example: linking risk controls to specifications, complaint codes to hazardous situations, and service findings to risk assessments.

Why this matters: Accessibility is the first prerequisite for accountability.

Build Defined Handoff Protocols Into Every Risk-Relevant Process

Every procedure that interacts with the risk management file — design transfer, change control, complaints, service records, PMS, management review, etc. — must include a defined, traceable step linking the activity to the risk management file.

Not a checkbox. Not a vague instruction to "consider risk." A specific, required connection. And more importantly, this must not be thought of as an operational burden.

Why this matters: Handoffs fail when risk is an afterthought. They succeed when risk is built into the process.

Invest in Cross-Functional Risk Management Competence

This is not a one-time training session. It is a long-term investment in organizational capability to help understand how risk flows through the device lifecycle, where each decision intersects with patient safety, and how to apply rigor commensurate with risk.

The Conversation the Book Has Been Building Toward

The twenty-plus functions described in this book are not the problem. Each has genuine expertise and genuine commitment to patient safety. The problem is that their contributions are not reliably connected — that the risk management file does not consistently receive what each function knows, and that each function does not consistently have access to or awareness of the risk management file.

Solving this is not primarily a technical challenge. Systems can connect data. The real challenge is organizational: **deciding that making risk management a connected capability is worth the sustained investment it requires**.

The patient who uses your device does not know which function bears responsibility for safety decisions. They experience the outcome of all of them. Risk management fails or succeeds as a system — as a set of connected contributions from every function working with a shared understanding of what patient safety requires and a shared commitment to make it possible.

Connecting these handoffs is not only a procedural task — it is a leadership responsibility.

Chapter 31: Building a Risk-Aware Organization

A risk-aware organization is built one decision at a time — and every decision begins with a mindset. Not a procedure. Not a checklist. A mindset.

It is the mindset that says: *patient safety is not someone else's job*. It is mine.

This book has shown how more than twenty functions across a medical device organization touch the risk management file. But the deeper message is this: **every function touches the patient**. Some directly. Some indirectly. Some visibly. Some quietly. But all meaningfully.

A risk-aware organization is not one where everyone becomes a risk expert. It is one where everyone understands their connection to patient safety — what they contribute to it, what decisions they make that affect it, and when they must pause and ask whether a choice they are about to make could harm the person who will one day use the device.

What This Looks Like in Practice

In a risk-aware organization, conversations sound different.

Design reviews include questions about whether specifications are safety-critical. Management reviews ask what complaint data reveals about real-world device risk. Post-market teams recognize that every code, every report, every observation is a link in the chain that keeps the risk management file honest.

But the transformation goes deeper than meetings.

It shows up in the quiet, unseen moments — the engineer who double-checks a requirement because she knows it is tied to a risk control; the complaint handler who adds one more detail because it might matter; the service technician who documents an unusual wear pattern because it could signal a failure mode not yet captured.

And it shows up in other corners of the organization too. A regulatory professional who pauses before submitting a labeling change and asks, *"Does this wording fully reflect the clinical consequence?"* A manufacturing technician who notices a subtle shift in a process parameter and flags it because they know it could affect device performance.

These are not procedural acts. They are acts of professional conscience.

Why This Matters

Because behind every requirement, every test, every complaint, every service call, every decision — there is a patient.

A real person. Someone who trusts that the device in their hands, on their body, or supporting their life is safe.

Most of the people whose lives you protect will never know your name. But they will feel the impact of your decisions.

Few industries place human life so directly in our hands. That is both a privilege and a responsibility.

What a Risk-Aware Organization Feels Like

A risk-aware organization has a center of gravity — a shared sense of purpose that guides decisions even when no one is watching. It feels like a place where:

- People speak up early, not late.
- Safety questions are welcomed, not avoided.
- Information flows freely across functions.
- Teams slow down when something feels wrong.
- Leaders model the behaviors they expect.
- The patient is present in every conversation, even when not named.

It feels like a place where the organization's "true north" is unmistakable: **the safety of the person who will one day rely on the device**.

A risk-aware organization is not built by policy. It is built by people.

How Culture Is Built

Culture does not emerge spontaneously. It is built — deliberately, consistently, and over time.

It is built through training that gives people the language of safety. Through systems that make risk-based thinking visible. Through cross-functional collaboration that breaks down silos. Through leaders who model the behaviors they expect. And through the accumulation of thousands of small decisions made with integrity.

Culture is built by what leaders pay attention to. But it is sustained by what individuals choose to do.

What This Means for You

At the center of a risk-aware culture is a simple question — one that does not require expertise in ISO 14971, only honesty: **How do my decisions affect the safety of the patient who will use this device?**

If every function asked this question consistently, the organization would already be risk-aware. All that remains is the structure that ensures the question is asked, that the right data is available to answer it, and that the answer flows to the right people at the right time.

This book has been an attempt to contribute to that structure — to give every function, every level of experience, and every professional in the medical device ecosystem the clarity they need to understand their role in patient safety.

Whether you are an entry-level engineer or a seasoned leader, your work shapes the safety of the devices that you help bring into the world.

A Final Call to Action

Risk management exists because patient trust must be earned — every day, through the quality of every decision we make.

So, as you close this book, carry forward this single truth:

Patient safety is not the responsibility of a department. It is the responsibility of an entire organization — including you.

Every role matters. Every decision matters. Every person matters.

Carry this responsibility with pride, with humility, and with the unwavering commitment that every patient deserves.

This is how a risk-aware organization is built — not through grand gestures, but through the steady, collective commitment of people who choose, again and again, to put the patient at the center of their work.

Leadership sets the tone. Culture is built by the choices each person makes.

And the patient — always — is why those choices matter.

www.ingramcontent.com/pod-product-compliance
Lightning Source LLC
LaVergne TN
LVHW010645110826
845149LV00014B/2958

* 9 7 9 8 9 9 5 9 8 0 4 9 0 *